P9-CQA-392

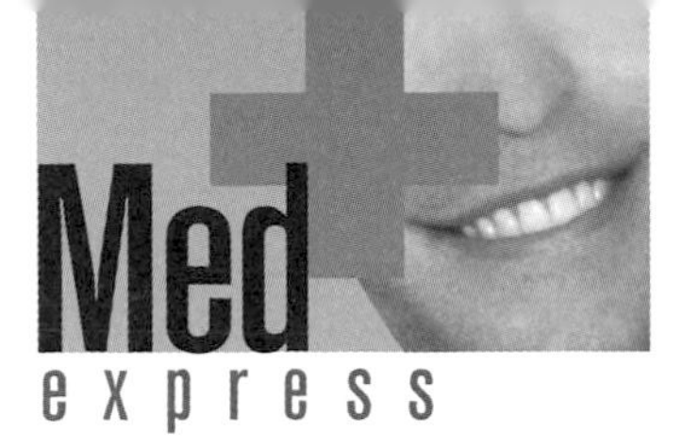

overcoming female discomforts

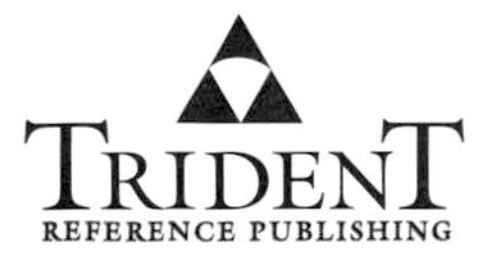

NOTE
This publication is intended to provide reference information for the reader on the covered subject. It is not intended to replace personalized medical diagnosis, counseling, and treatment from a doctor or other healthcare professional.
Before taking any form of treatment you should always consult your physician or medical practitioner.
The publisher and authors disclaim any liability, loss, injury or damage incurred as a consequence, directly or indirectly, of the use and application of the contents of this book.

Published by:
Trident Reference Publishing
801 12th Avenue South, Suite 400
Naples, Fl 34102 USA
Phone: + 1 239 649 7077
Email: sales@trident-international.com
Website: www.trident-international.com

Overcoming Female Discomforts

Publisher
Simon St. John Bailey

Editor-in-chief
Isabel Toyos

Art Director
Aline Talavera

Photos
© Trident Reference Publishing, © Getty Images,
© Jupiter Images, © Planstock, © J. Alonso

Includes index
ISBN 1582799733 (hc)
UPC 615269997338 (hc)
ISBN 158279961X (pbk)
UPC 615269799611 (pbk)

2005 Edition
Printed in USA

overcoming female discomforts

What are female discomforts?

Women's reproductive organs make up a complex system that may cause various female discomforts at different stages of life. Knowing what these discomforts are and their causes may help you to identify the simple symptoms that affect your body and to know when to visit your doctor for a professional diagnosis.

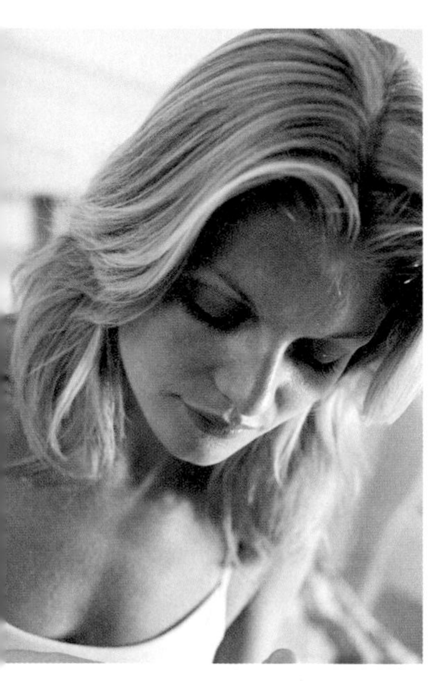

Women's bodies, when fertilized during conception, become pregnant and can give birth to a child. The female reproductive system undergoes cyclical events. The reproductive cycle begins with the ovaries, releasing female egg cells called ova into the Fallopian tubes. Conception, normally occurs in the fallopian tubes. After conception, the uterus becomes the environment for the fertilized egg or zygote. The zygote can grow into an embryo and after three months of pregnancy, a fetus. The fetus continues to grow inside the uterus until the baby travels through the birth canal on the way to being born.

The ovaries not only produce ova; they also produce the female sex hormones progesterone and estrogen. Other hormones secreted by the pituitary gland, interact with the hormones produced by the ovaries, to maintain the reproductive and menstrual cycle. Ovulation takes place on, or around the 14th day of the menstrual cycle. If the mature ovum is fertilized, conception occurs; if the egg is not fertilized, it is discharged with the lining of the womb, this process constitutes the menstruation period. Each woman's menstrual cycle varies from puberty until menopause. Your period is affected by hormonal changes caused by pregnancy, childbirth, age, nervous states or illnesses. These fluctuations can cause a number of discomforts, such as premenstrual syndrome (PMS), abundant hemorrhaging, irregular or few periods and other irregularities. Menopause is also associated with a number of discomforts, not limited to this stage of life, such as hot flashes, osteoporosis and vaginal drying. During pregnancy normal discomforts include morning sickness, backaches and trouble sleeping.

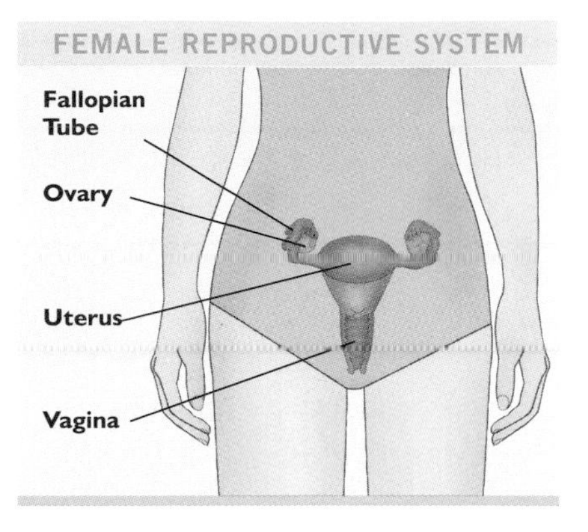

Breast problems, vaginal yeast infections and other ailments can appear at any stage of a woman's life. All of these discomforts can affect your energy, making you tired or depressed. You should always visit your doctor to treat any female discomfort. In addition, there are a number of complementary therapies that can help to relieve symptoms and fortify the immune system.

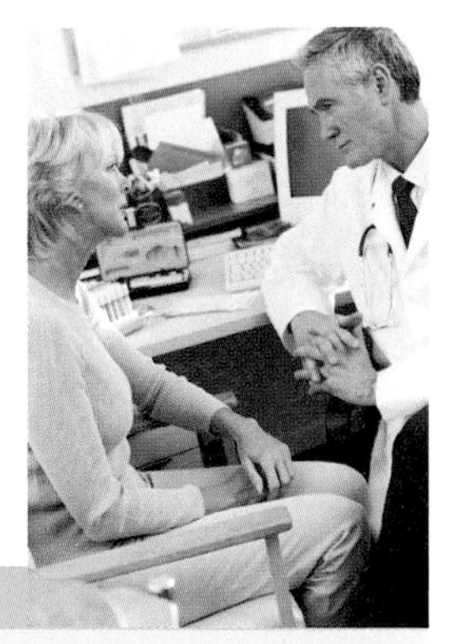

ANNUAL TESTS

Gynecological tests, should be a regular practice from puberty throughout adult womanhood. You should visit your gynecologist at least once a year for a check-up. Women who are susceptible to infections, or with history of breast or ovarian cancer should visit their gynecologist every 6 months. Tests done during a routine check-up:

- **Smears Test**
- **Pelvic Examination**
- **External Genital Examination**
- **Speculum Examination**
- **Breast Examination**
- **Mammography** Women over 40 should have mammograms every year; younger women whose families have a history of breast cancer should consult their clinicians.
- **Densitometric Analysis or Bone Density Test** During menopause.

Frequent symptoms

Women can suffer from many, diverse discomforts during their reproductive lives. Symptoms vary with age and for each person. We've put together a guide for the most common problems and symptoms.

Healthy as you may be, you may from time to time experience discomforts related to your reproductive system. However, the healthier you keep your body and lifestyle, the better you may overcome these discomforts which can cause problems for most women.

PREMENSTRUAL SYNDROME (PMS)

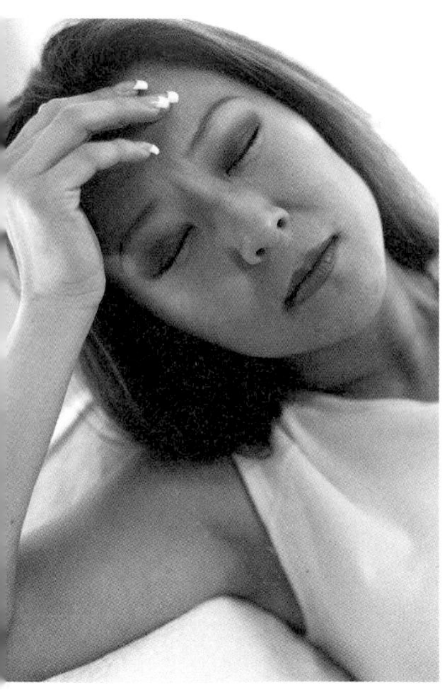

There's hardly a woman on the planet who doesn't know the misery of period pains. Premenstrual syndrome is a number of symptoms related to the menstrual cycle, occuring 5 to 11 days before you begin to menstruate and disappearing shortly after. Surveys show that 75 percent of young women regularly uses painkillers to cope with the pain and at least 50 percent says it seriously disrupts their lives.

The most common symptoms are caused by the hormones released and include: anxiety, sweating, increased heart rate, dizziness, headaches, cramps, insomnia and fatigue. Symptoms can also bring on a number of emotional or mental states such as depression, apathy, fear, aggression and confusion, or organic symptoms such as over-sensitive breasts, bloating or weight gain and acne breakouts.

DURING PREGNANCY

Pregnancy causes a number of changes in women's bodies, these are frequently accompanied by ailments and discomforts such as:

- Nausea, heartburn, changes in appetite.
- Anaemia.
- Backaches and neck aches.
- Headaches and migraines.
- Constipation, hemorrhoids, and varicose veins.
- Cramped legs.
- Changes in sleep pattern, stress and anxiety.

BREAST DISCOMFORTS

Many women, from the age of puberty suffer changes due to hormonal activity as well as hereditary and diet factors. Although the majority of breast discomforts tend to be benign, some deserve special consideration. If you suffer from any symptom you should consult your gynecologist.

■ **Breast pain.** It's also known as "mastalgia." Breast pain may occur in one or both breasts or in the underarm (axilla) region of the body. The severity of breast pain varies from woman to woman.

■ **Lumps.** Breast lumps are abnormal hard formations that are sometimes detected with breast examinations. They may be benign formations, but if you detect a lump you should consult your doctor immediately.

■ **Mastitis.** It's a relatively common problem for breast-feeding mothers; sometimes, mastitis may be caused by the breast becoming over-full, or blocked because of milk over-supply, ineffective breastfeeding, missed feeds, restrictive clothing or bruising. Although mastitis can be caused by a number of factors, you should consult your doctor for the correct treatment.

SYMPTOM DIARY

It's recommended that you keep a "symptom diary" for at least three months, to know which symptoms relate to your menstrual cycle. This log book may help your doctor not only to more precisely diagnose PMS, but also help your physician to choose the most appropriate treatment.

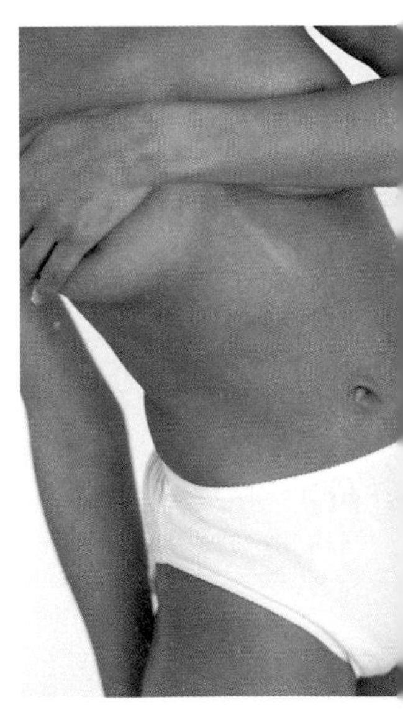

■ **Nipple discharge.** Frequent in women over the age of 30, this is generally caused by hormonal changes. Nipple discharge is any type of fluid or secretion emanating from the nipple or the areola. Any woman with a suspicious or worrisome nipple discharge should consult her physician.

■ **Breast cysts.** Simple cysts are typically round or oval and have smooth edges. Breast cysts, tiny accumulations of fluid, which contain a viscous liquid that makes cysts feel hard. The size varies. If you detect a formation you should consult your physician immediately.

BREAST SELF-EXAMINATION

Women who are menstruating should perform a breast examination 7 to 10 days after menstruation, when the breasts are less sensitive. For women who are no longer menstruating or are breastfeeding, it's best to perform this exam the same day of every month.

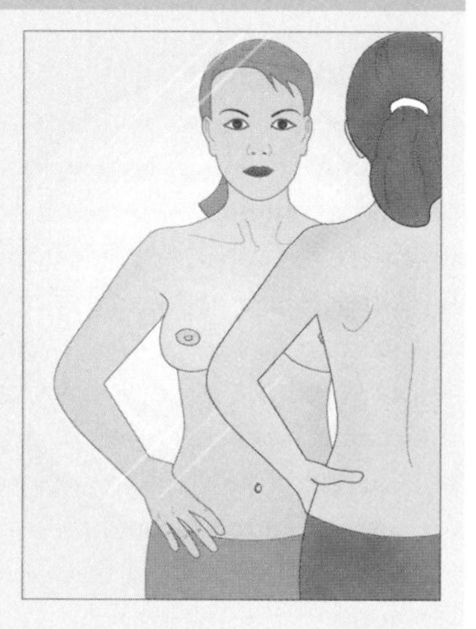

1. Stand in front of a mirror. Place your hands on your hips and press firmly inward, tightening your chest muscles, while looking at your breasts for any change in their usual appearance. Perform leaning slightly forward and again while standing upright. Next, pressing both hands behind your head, look for changes in the shape and size of your breasts.

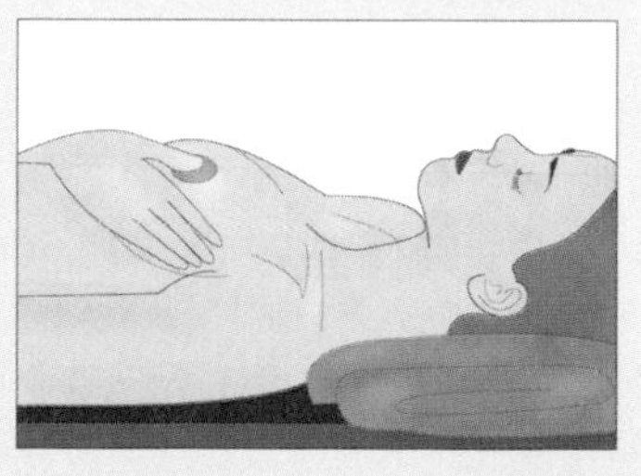

2. Lying down. To examine your left breast, lie flat on your back with a pillow or folded towel under your left shoulder. Raise your left arm over your head. Use the flat portions of the second, third and fourth fingertips of your right hand to examine your left breast. Press gently to feel tissues under the skin and then more firmly for deep tissues. Repeat for the right breast. If you detect any change, it's important that you visit your health care provider immediately.

CANDIDIASIS

Candidiasis is a common infection caused by a type of yeast-like fungus called candida. Yeast infections are common for women who are taking birth control pills containing estrogen and for pregnant women. Hormonal changes can also bring on yeast infections. Sometimes antibiotics or medicines can contribute to the growth of candida. Symptoms usually include:

- Abnormal white, thick and lumpy discharge.
- Itching and/or burning in the vaginal labia and in the vagina.
- Vulvar redness and swelling.
- Discomfort during or after sexual intercourse.
- Pain or burning when passing urine.

PAY ATTENTION TO ABNORMAL BLEEDING

If you notice any vaginal bleeding outside of the normal menstrual cycle, or abnormally heavy bleeding during menstruation, you should consult your gynecologist inmediately. The same applies even more urgently to any loss of blood at any stage of the nine months of pregnancy.

MENOPAUSE

Menopause is a period of transition, the time at "mid-life" when a woman ceases to menstruate. It happens when the ovaries begin to stop releasing eggs –usually a gradual process, although sometimes it happens all at once. The ovaries' production of female hormones (estrogen and progesterone) slows down during this stage. Menopause is a natural physical occurrence for women, usually between the ages of 40 and 55. Some women experience few symptoms or none, while others suffer from a series of symptoms, varying from slight to severe:

- Hot flashes.
- Loss of energy.
- Changes in sexual desire.
- Irregular menstrual periods or periods that stop.
- Vaginal dryness and discomfort during sexual relations.
- Changes in the skin's appearance and the mucous membranes.

Fighting discomforts

Many female discomforts are natural and often times they influence the way women feel emotionally and mentally. There are some natural alternative remedies that can provide relief. However, if you find that the discomforts become abnormal, or you notice sores or infections you should visit your doctor immediately.

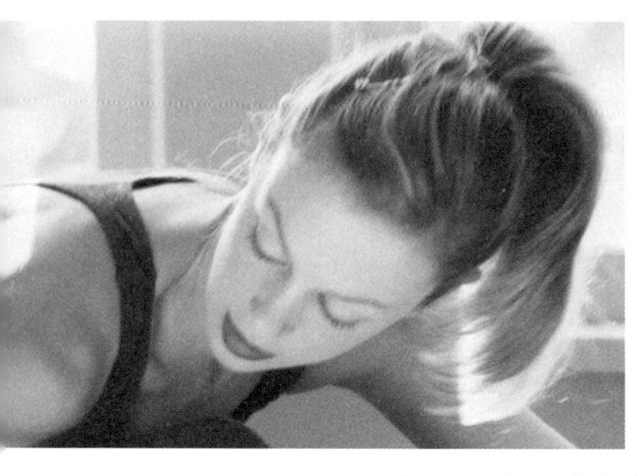

A healthy diet and regular exercise can be a good way to start you off on the right track to relieving some female discomforts.

Healthy diet. It's recommended that you reduce your coffee, tea, salt, sugar, fat and alcohol consumption. At the same time you should make sure you drink an ample amount of water (at least 6 to 8 glasses per day). Also, it is especially important for women to make sure they eat calcium rich foods daily throughout their entire life: it's important to eat at least three to five portions daily (one portion of calcium is equivalent to 1 glass of milk, 1 piece of cheese or 1 yogurt). This habit should begin during infancy, reinforced during pregnancy and while breastfeeding. It's important to get enough calcium throughout women's adulthood to prevent osteoporosis and to protect the bones.

HEALTH AFTER 50

Lack of estrogen causes the cells that build new bone to be less active than the cells that remove old bone. Your bones are being depleted faster than they are being built up. The excessive loss of bone mass causes osteoporosis, a thinning and weakening of the bones. Lack of estrogen also causes changes in your cholesterol levels, and puts you at higher risk of diseases.

■ **Good habits.** It's important to quit smoking. Getting enough physical exercise, which hardens and helps to fix calcium in the bones, is also very important, as is keeping your stress levels to a minimum.

IMPORTANCE OF ACCEPTANCE

Through all the physical changes throughout women's lives it's important to keep a positive outlook and to accept the changes. Admitting that during each menstruation PMS causes you to become irritable, accepting that after childbirth it's natural for women to go through a brief bout of depression or learning to get over the side effects of menopause, an accepting and tolerant attitude will help you to better overcome your female discomforts. In all cases, it may be helpful to get psychological help, in the form of individual or group therapy. It can be helpful to share your mental symptoms and the anxieties brought on by these physical changes to better manage the symptoms; especially those brought on by hormonal changes.

WARNING

These symptoms of female discomforts are the most common. However, bear in mind that there are many other discomforts and illnesses not listed, which can present slight to serious symptoms and physical side effects. The content of this book is provided for general information only, and should not be treated as a substitute for the medical advice of your own doctor or any other health care professional. You should get an annual or bi-annual gynecological check up to make sure that your symptom is not caused by a serious physical defect.

NATURAL HELP

There are several alternative medicines and therapies that are said to be helpful in the treatment of the symptoms of menopause, including:

- Aromatherapy and essential oils used in baths, massages and self-massages.
- Herbal medicine, including herbs that contain phytoestrogens, ideal for menopause.
- Hydrotherapy.
- Yoga.
- Reflexology.
- *Shiatsu*.

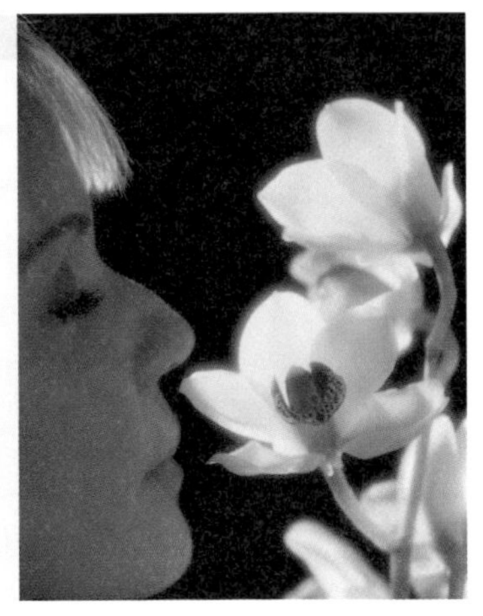

Relaxation techniques

The following simple and easy-to-do techniques can be excellent in helping to relieve the discomforts associated with PMS, pregnancy and menopause.

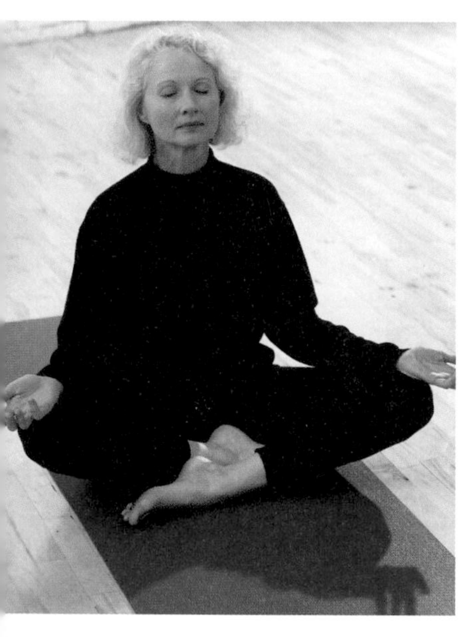

As female discomforts directly affect mood swings and increase stress and nervous states, relaxation is a key factor in relieving symptoms.

BREATHING AND RELIEF

The process of breathing is fundamental for relieving any kind of pain. Deep and even breathing can help to relax the muscles, slow down the heart rate and temporarily lower blood pressure. It also helps to calm the mind, generating the alpha brain waves associated with deep relaxation. There are many different breathing exercises; one of the most appropriate for calming agitated moods is the following:

- **Alternate, balanced breathing.** Ideal for relaxing and fighting depressive states associated with PMS and menopause. In a comfortable position, either lying down or sitting, begin to breathe through each of the nostrils.

1. Place your index and middle fingers on the bridge of your nose. While you block your nostril with your thumb, inhale counting to four; next, exhale counting to four.
2. Continue by relaxing your thumb and cover your other nostril with your ring finger. Inhale and exhale 4 times. You can repeat this

exercise 10 times on each side and as you continue practicing you can increase the amount of time progressively.

EXERCISING AGAINST TENSION

This exercise is very useful for relaxing tension and releasing anxiety especially in PMS, pregnancy and menopause.

1. Lying on your back, with your legs stretched out and your arms to your side. With your eyes closed, take a deep breath eight times. Hold your breath in four seconds and exhale in eight seconds.

2. In the same position, lift up your knees and place your feet on the ground, hip width apart. Repeat the previous breathing exercise. When you inhale, imagine that your body is filling with energy; when you exhale imagine that your body is getting rid of tiredness, pain and anxiety. Repeat this exercise three times, very slowly.

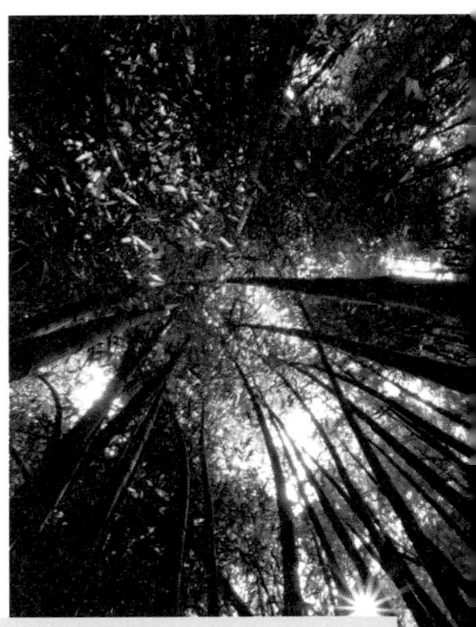

CREATIVE VISUALIZATION

This type of visualization uses the power of positive thought and the imagination to create or recreate an image or an ideal situation and to experience positive emotions. It is very useful for reaching a relaxed state of general well-being, for helping you "erase" negative emotions such as fear or anger. This technique is recommended for pregnant women to connect with their baby in the womb.
In all cases, this exercise begins with conscious breathing, inhaling and exhaling slowly. Next, visualize a beautiful landscape in which you can relax and breathe deeply.

- **To get rid of negative thoughts.** Visualize a blue sky with floating clouds. As you inhale connect with that negative thought or feeling and as you exhale place it on the cloud, allowing it to float away each time you exhale.
- **For pregnant women.** Sitting with your hands on your chest, visualize your child and generate positive thoughts and images of your future together.

Exercising to relieve aches

One of the best ways to relax the body and mind –a basic treatment for female discomforts– is physical exercise. A guide with the exercises specifically recommended for pregnant women and women undergoing menopause hass been put together for you.

Physical exercise helps to regulate neuroendocrine activity and blood circulation and helps in the distribution of minerals in the bones. Before starting any exercise program, it's recommended:

- Consult your doctor and have a medical checkup.
- Don't eat during the two hours before exercising.
- Always warm up for 20 minutes (exercise bike, cycling or walking) to prevent injuries.
- Use comfortable cotton clothing and good sports shoes.

10 GOOD REASONS FOR WORKING OUT

1. Fortifies your immune system.
2. Decreases your risk of cardiovascular disease.
3. Improves your mood and humor.
4. Improves your sleep and mental clarity.
5. Keeps your weight under control, not only your weight is lowered with regular exercise, your anxiety is lowered and your appetite is regulated.
6. Fights against headaches and backaches.
7. Increases the level of HDL or "good cholesterol" in your blood system.
8. Strengthens your bones and helps to prevent osteoporosis.
9. Increases your muscular resistance and mass, which improves your balance and prevents injuries and broken bones.
10. Prevents type II diabetes (adult diabetes).

MUSCLE RELAXING EXERCISES

Before and during menstruation, our bodies tend to build up nervous tension particularly in the shoulders and neck, making us feel achy and heavy. To release tension these simple, loosening exercises may also be beneficial during menopause and pregnancy.

Shoulders

Sitting with your back straight and your arms relaxed to your sides, gently roll your shoulders forward and backward, slowly and smoothly.

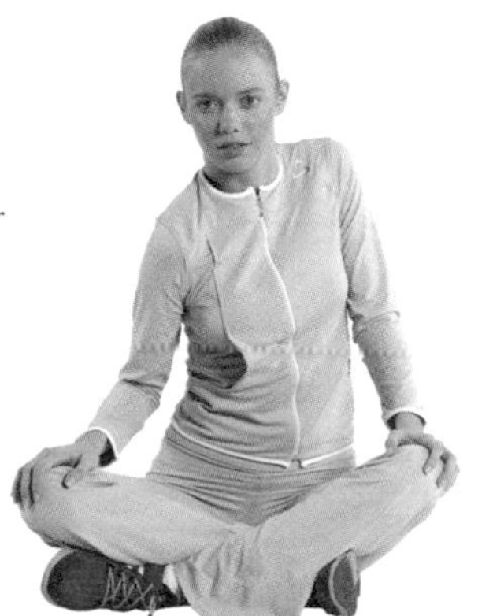

NOTE
Every woman requires a different type of training according to her age and physical state. Before starting any exercise program it is important that you visit your doctor for a physical checkup so that he or she can recommend appropriate exercises, how often you should do them and if you need to take any special precautions.

Neck

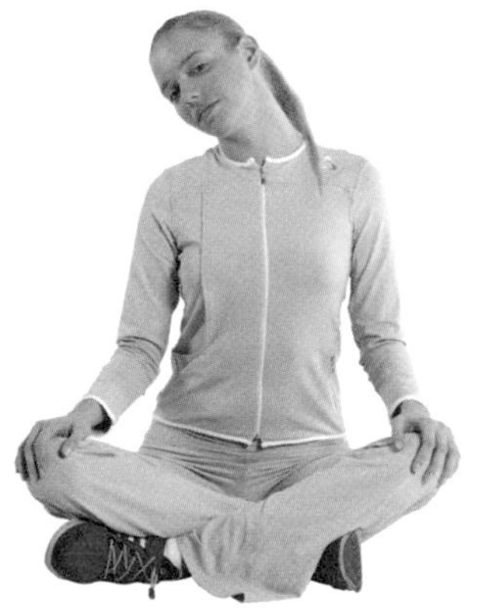

1. *Sitting with your legs crossed, hands on your knees and back straight, roll your head in slow circular movements, five times to the right and five to the left, breathing deeply and slowly as you perform the exercise.*

2. *Start with your head centered and facing forward, gently move your head backward only to where it's comfortable. Breathe in and hold your breath; then, breathe out. Concentrate on how your neck feels as it stretches and your throat zone opens.*

DURING PREGNANCY

• It's recommended that you continue with a regular exercise routine during pregnancy because it provides a number of benefits: increases your energy, keeps and improves blood circulation and flexibility. It also improves your posture, increases your awareness of your body and your physical movements. Walking, swimming and aqua aerobics are recommended exercises.

• During pregnancy you should avoid high impact aerobic exercises, involving jumping or running and contact sports such as hockey or volleyball. At the same time, it's best that you consult your doctor before exercising during pregnancy.

• **Swimming and aqua aerobics.** Swimming is an excellent sport during pregnancy, it doesn't involve any risk, because muscular exercises in the water don't involve impact or joint resistance. It improves your breathing and keeps your muscles toned and your joints flexible. You should avoid very cold or hot water; appropriate temperature is between 77 to 90°F/25 to 32°C.

• **Walking.** Walking is a great way to keep your muscles toned, improve your blood circulation and breathing and keep your cardiovascular system healthy, without straining your body.

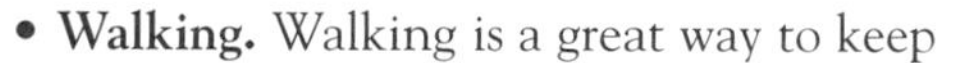

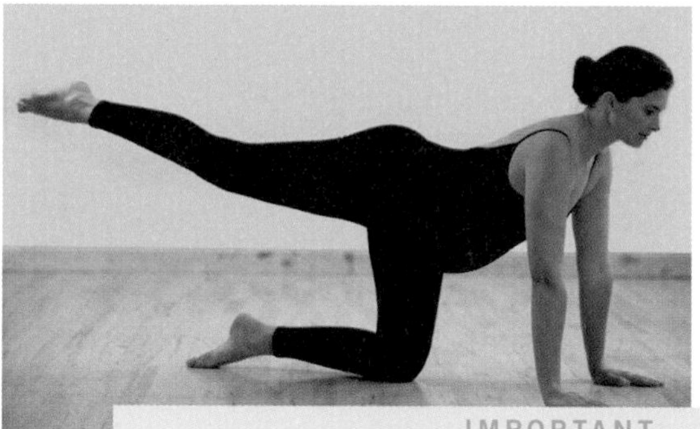

EXERCISE AND PREGNANCY

Not every type of exercise is appropriate during pregnancy. Weight training and aerobics classes are not advised, even if you were regularly practicing them before getting pregnant. Recommended workouts include stretching, yoga, rhythmic dance and classical ballet, but they should be practiced moderately and using caution.

IMPORTANT

When you are working out during pregnancy you should keep in mind:

- Your pulse shouldn't go over 140 beats per minute. Never do intense exercises for more than 15 minutes at a time.
- Avoid any exercises involving rolling, jumping or bouncing.
- If you experience any pain or complications, stop exercising and immediately visit your obstetrician.
- Don't overheat your body.

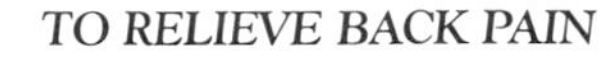

TO RELIEVE BACK PAIN

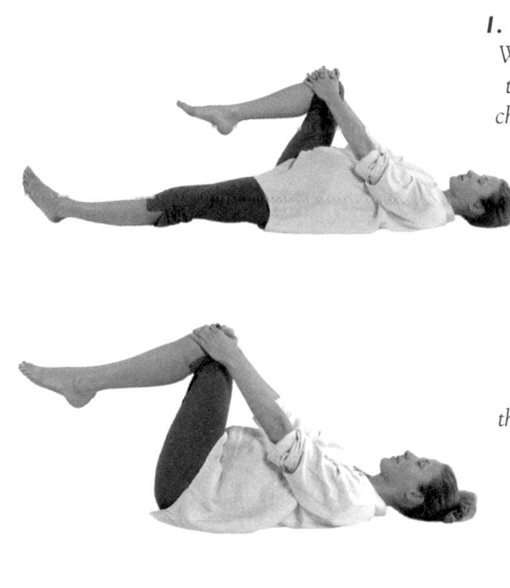

1. Lie on the floor on your back. With one leg stretched out, and the other with the knee to your chest. Wrap your hands around your knee and hug your leg into your chest. Stay in this position for a few minutes and then repeat with the other leg.

2. Lie down in the same position, bring both of your knees to your chest and hug them. Stay in this position for a few minutes and then relax. Practice these exercises for as long as you feel comfortable. Never strain or use force.

DURING MENOPAUSE

• It's been proven that after 40 years-old our bodies begin to lose muscular mass; making walking, biking, swimming or rowing the most recommended aerobic exercises for this age group. It's important for your body to make weight bearing movements, to strengthen the bones, especially in the hips. You should do any of these exercises at least three times a week.

• If you suffer from osteoporosis, a low-risk activity is biking on an exercise bike, to avoid falling and possible broken bones.

• It's best to increase the time and rhythm as you build your stamina over time. Over exerting yourself during a high impact or intense exercises may cause injuries, muscle cramps or sprains. It's not recommended that you participate in sports involving jumping, running or races.

SPEED WALKING

When you start out its best to use a moderate pace and then build up your stamina for a few months before speed walking. If you haven't exercised in a while, start with a 10 to 12 minute walk, adding a minute per week, until you build up to an hour three times a week. After walking it's important that you stretch out to avoid muscular pains and to improve your flexibility. You can use your arms while walking; over time you can add hand weights of between 2 and 4 pounds.

Harmonizing yoga

In Sanskrit means *harmonizing your body, spirit and mind.* Yoga exercises work on all the various systems of the body and provide a number of benefits for women; helping to relieve discomforts brought on by menstruation, pregnancy and menopause.

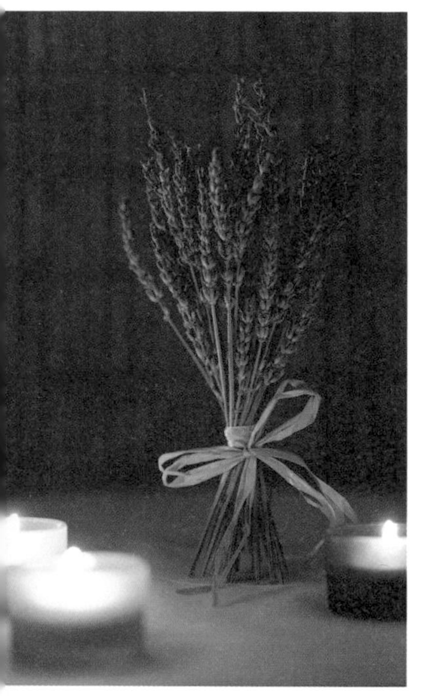

✚ During the different cycles of the menstrual periods, pregnancy and menopause, women undergo an important number of changes in the production of estrogen, progesterone and calcium metabolizing. There are a number of yoga poses that help to balance these functions, helping to maintain bone density. Also, they help to regulate ovary function and hypothalamus and pituitary glands, which control the endocrine system, generating menopause.

THE COBRA

This *asana* is beneficial for the female body because it regulates the suprarenal glands' function and strengthens the

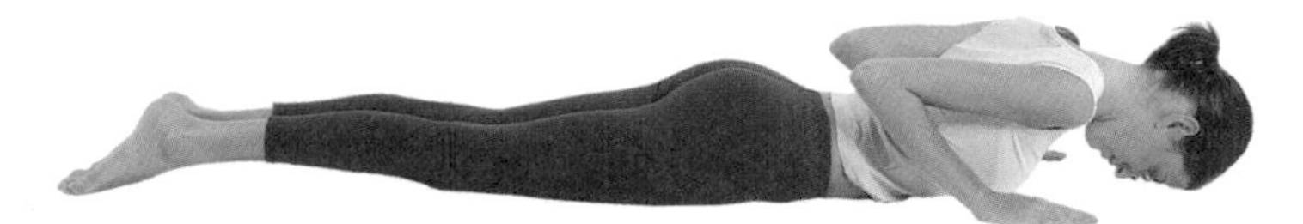

1. *Lie down with your legs together and your forehead rested on the palms of your hands on the floor. Your legs should be straight with the front of your feet resting on the floor. Press your buttocks to help you move into the next position and place your elbows, forearms and the palms of your hands on the floor. Your elbows should stay at the same height as your shoulders and your head pressed against the floor.*

back, increases the flexibility of the spine and helps to tone the abdominal muscles. In addition, it helps to increase your energy and to lift up your self-esteem. It helps to regulate your menstrual period and relieves tension, but it shouldn't be practiced while you are menstruating.

2. *Lift up your chest, always with your buttocks contracted. So as not to harm the neck, extend your arms at the same time as you lift up your chest. If this causes any discomfort, don't strain yourself and keep your head looking forward. Breathe normally. To release, slowly lower your body while you place on the ground (in this order): the abdomen, the chest and lastly the chin, always stretched forward. Next, bring your chin downward and rest one cheek on the ground.*

SHOULDER STAND

This *asana* is recommended for discomforts caused by premenstrual syndrome, because it regulates blood circulation throughout the body, relieving tension and pain. Do not practice this pose while you are menstruating.

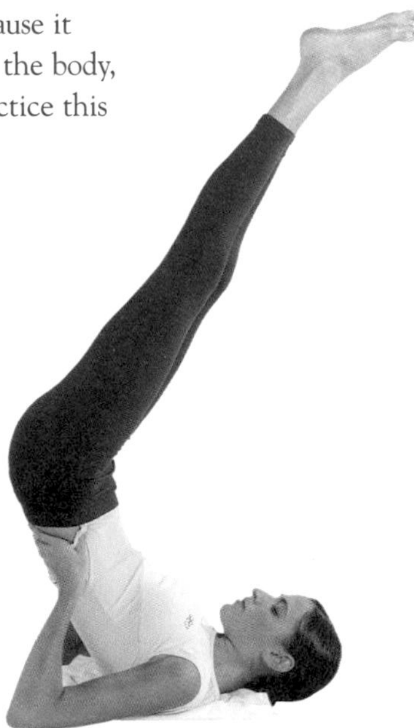

Lie down on the floor with your legs together and your hands, palms down, by your sides. Inhaling, push down on your hands and raise your legs straight up above you; exhale. As you inhale lift your hips off the floor and bring your legs up, over and beyond your head, at an angle of about 45 degrees. Exhaling, bend your arms and support your body, holding as near the shoulders as possible, thumbs around the front of the body, fingers around the back. Push your back up, try to lift your legs to a near vertical position. Stay in this position for as long as you feel comfortable, breathing slowly and deeply in the pose.

CAT POSE

This *asana* is ideal to help relieve abdominal pain during PMS and your period. It is also ideal for pains during pregnancy.

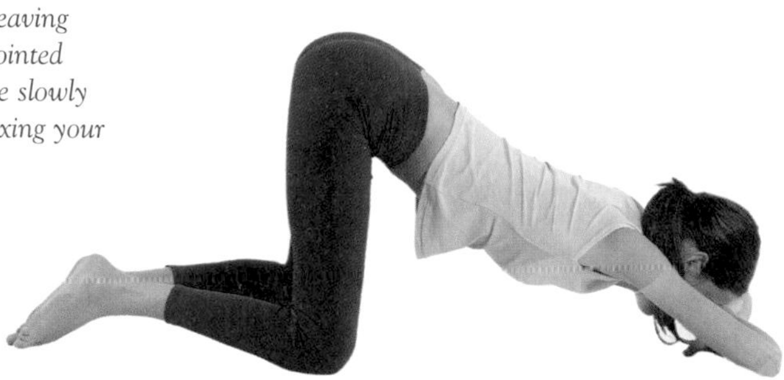

Start on your hands and knees, with your knees fully spread. Move your hips back, fold your arms and place your forehead on your arms, leaving your buttocks pointed upward. Breathe slowly and deeply, relaxing your entire body.

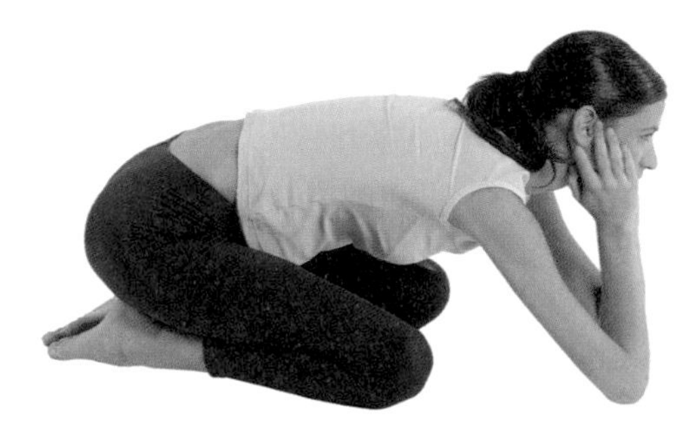

Another variation that may be more comfortable and relieves pain. Start from the previous position, bring together your ankles and sit on them with your elbows pressed to the floor. Stay in this asana *for as long as you feel comfortable, breathing naturally and deeply, looking for maximum relaxation.*

YOGA FOR EVERY STAGE OF LIFE

- **For premenstrual syndrome and menstrual cramps.** During the first two days of menstruation, it's best to only do breathing and relaxation exercises. You should not do upside down poses while menstruating.
- **During pregnancy.** Yoga is a gentle way of keeping your body active and supple and minimizes the common pregnancy symptoms like morning sickness and constipation. As long as you aren't experiencing bleeding or any other medical complication, you can practice yoga

without problems during pregnancy. It also helps in restoring your body shape, uterus, abdomen, and pelvic floor, and in relieving upper back tension and breast discomfort after childbirth. The *Pranayama* breathing techniques can also become handy during labor, and improve circulation for mother and baby, helping both to relax. You should avoid poses that work the glandular parts of the body. Special care, however, is needed in choosing the yoga poses that you will practice, you should avoid poses that require an inverted position or laying on the belly.

• **During menopause.** This is one of the most beneficial physical exercises and the least risky. Practicing yoga after 50 years of age helps to keep you physically fit, mentally healthy and to avoid a sedentary lifestyle.

GENTLE EXERCISE

Yoga is a discipline designed to improve your flexibility and harmony. The exercises use gentle movements without straining your body. When practicing the *asanas* remember not to strain yourself. There is no need to push yourself too far. Remember to use gentle movements and don't push your body into a pose.

YOGA POSE FOR MENOPAUSE. THE TRIANGLE POSE

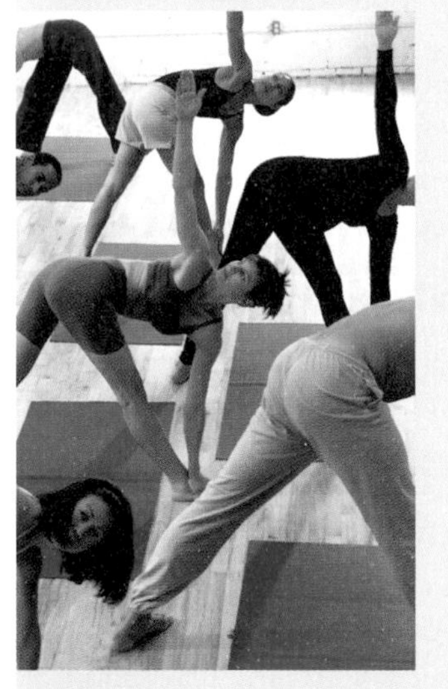

This is the asana most widely used in the prevention of osteoporosis. It's advised to practice this pose at any age, but especially during menopause. It gives an excellent lateral stretch to the spine, toning the spinal nerves and abdominal muscles. It also strengthens the legs, reducing the probability of a fractured hip. In addition, it balances your body, making the muscles and joints more flexible, especially in the pelvic region. If your body isn't very flexible, use a wall for extra support.

Safety. Do not practice this pose if you suffer from meniscus, herniated disk or hip problems.

1. Stand with your feet well apart. Raise your arms parallel to the floor and reach them to the sides, shoulder blades wide, palms down. Without bending your knees, extend your torso and turn your right foot out.

2. As you inhale, bend your torso to the right and bring both hands to your right ankle (or shin, depending on how flexible you are). Extend your right arm toward the ceiling with your palm facing away from you. Look out at your right hand. Take several full breaths in this position before releasing it. Release and repeat, bending to the other side.

Reflexology for her

Reflexology is an ancient healing art based on the principle that there are reflexes in the body –especially on the feet– that correspond to the body's organs and glands. Stimulating and applying pressure to the feet may be effective in helping relieve many symptoms of female discomforts.

DURING PREGNANCY

It is recommended to consult a reflexology specialist, especially if you've had incidence of miscarriage or a risky pregnancy.

Reflexology considers that using the rhythmic pressing of acupressure points for short periods, helps to unblock or to balance the flow of vital energy –or *chi*– to regulate energy imbalances that can provoke illnesses. The following exercises may help to relax your body and to restore your psychophysical balance in the face of the pains caused by PMS, pregnancy and menopause.

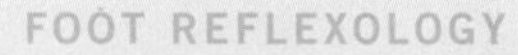

The basic areas for reflexology massages to help to overcome female discomforts are the following:

- **The bottom of the feet.** This area corresponds to the chest cavity, side of the neck, the spinal column, the sacrum, the thyroids and the suprarenal glands.
- **The outer edge of the foot.** The pelvic area and the ovaries.
- **The inner part of the foot.** The uterus and areas of the spinal column.

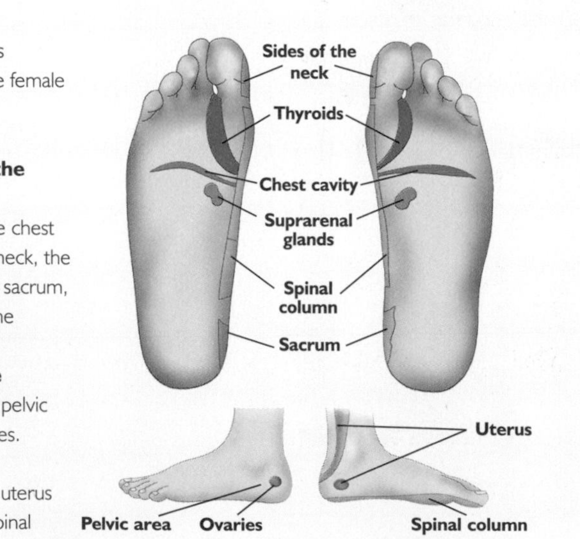

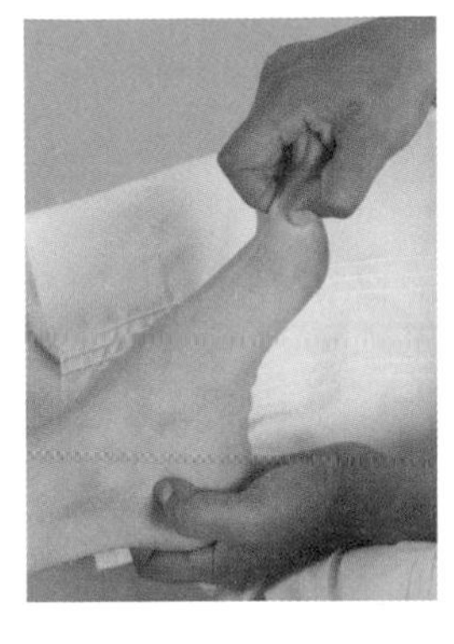

Tension in the neck

Massage the toes, on the joint that joins the toes to the foot; especially on the big toe that corresponds to the neck. Massage for 2-3 minutes.

Backache

Massage the arch of the foot, which corresponds to the spinal column. Use the thumbs to knead along the edge of the foot, using small circular motions from the ankle up to the toes.

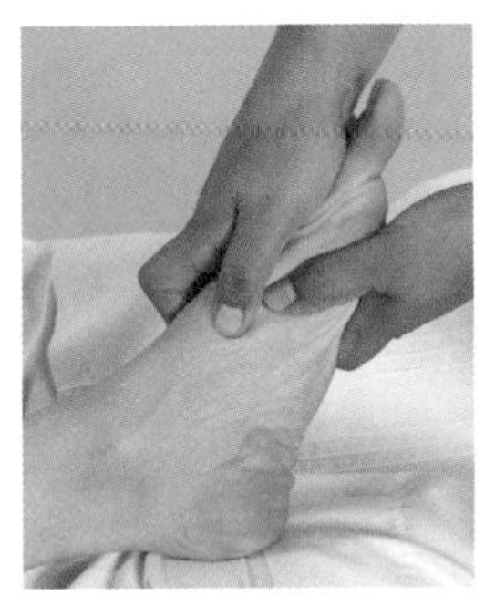

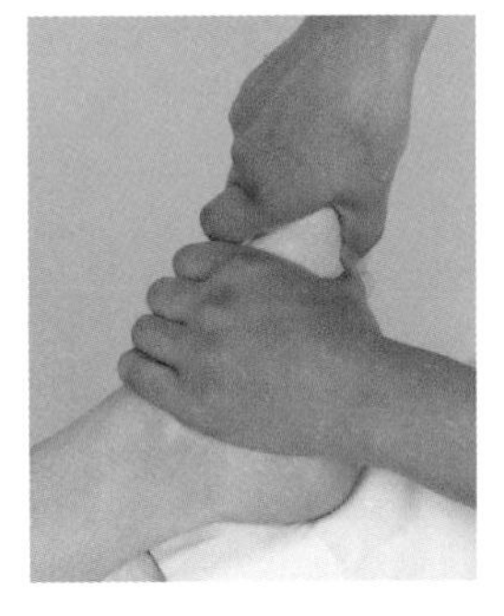

Calming your mind and emotions

Massage the bottom and the edges of the feet to relax and soothe the mind and emotions. Gently massage along the entire foot, especially in the mid and upper areas, including the toes. This is a great massage for over all well-being.

Premenstrual problems

To help fight discomforts associated with PMS, a week before your menstrual period starts:

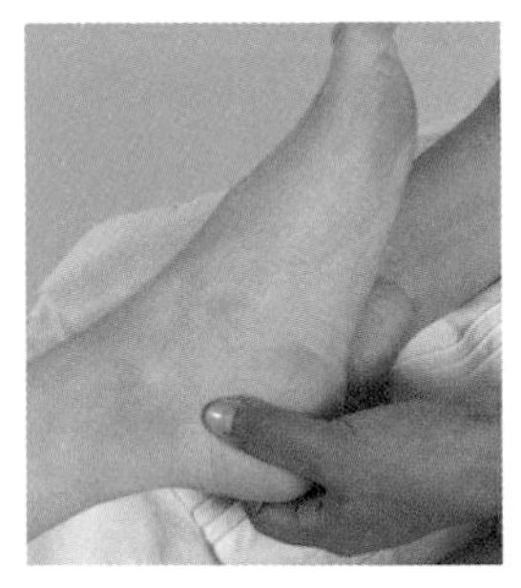

1. *Massage the areas that reflect the ovaries and pelvis.*

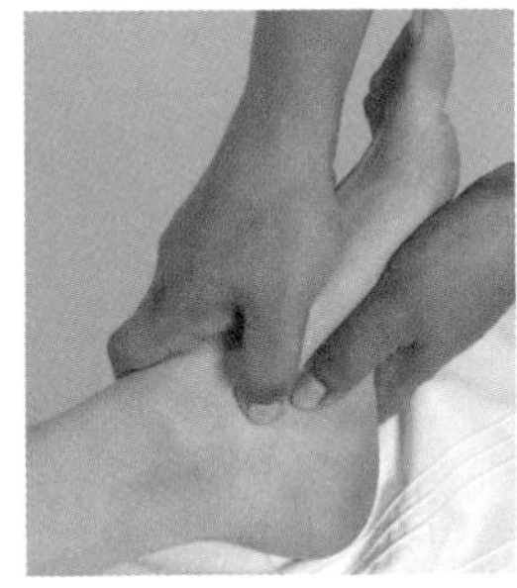

2. *Apply pressure on the point that reflects the lower back.*

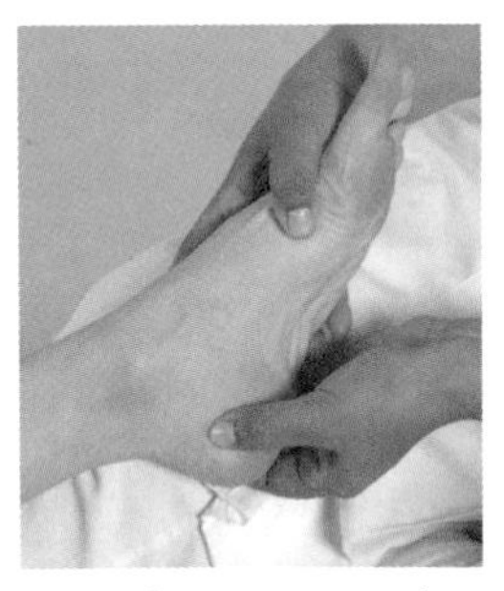

3. *Lastly, massage on the point that reflects the sacrum (the lowest point of the back) that is located close to the heel.*

Curing caresses

Giving yourself massages on specific areas is a great gift for your body and soul. Massages can help to release tension and relieve discomforts brought on by your menstrual period. They also help to pick up your energy. We've put together a guide of techniques ideal for the most difficult days.

According to the Chinese healing art *qi gong*, there is vital energy flowing through our bodies, circulating through special channels –or meridians– throughout the body. The discipline of *qi gong* consists of a series of gentle movements, without using muscular strength, to conserve and restore the body's energy.

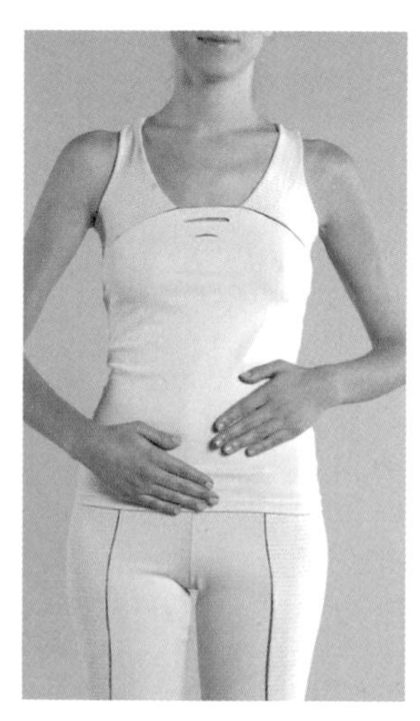

1. Place your hands on the dantian and rub using slanted and alternating movements (when one hand moves up the other lowers). Rub up and down 30 times.

FOR PMS

For PMS, menopause or postpartum apply massages on the dantian, the central point of the body, where vital energy is stored from where it's distributed. This point helps to restore balance and harmony for women.

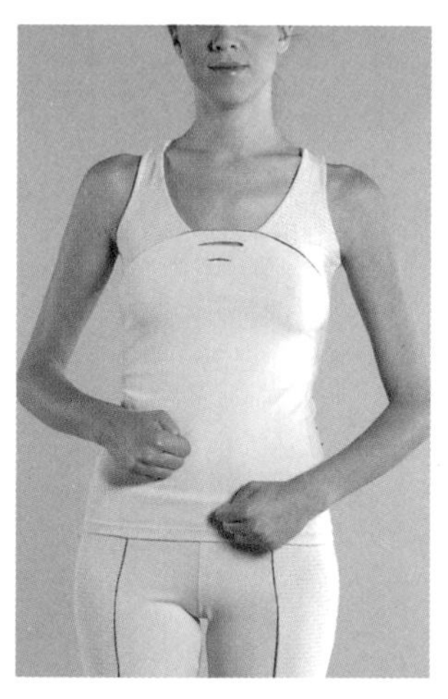

2. Next, close your fists and with your wrists relaxed apply gentle alternating taps with one fist at a time along the dantian, stimulating the distribution of energy along the meridians. Repeat 30 times with each fist.

AFTER CHILD BIRTH

The following massage is especially good for toning the abdominal muscles after giving birth.

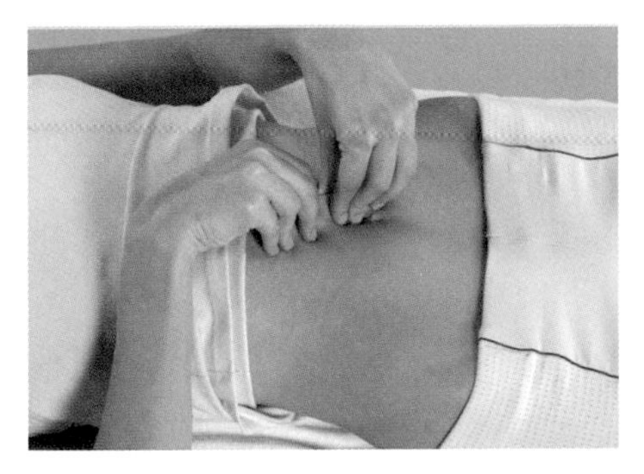

PAINFUL BREASTS

Gently massage the breasts with essential oil of lavender or geranium, diluted with a neutral oil, to relieve pains during breast milk production during the last months of pregnancy. This massage is also effective during the days before menstruation.

1. *Lie down on your back and with your fingers gently "pinch" the skin, lifting it up, pulling and then releasing.*

2. *Repeat the technique of lifting up the skin, but this time alternating with both hands. Continue the massage for a few minutes, alternating hands. Use the same technique on the other side. Next, slide the hands down to the muscles over the womb and continue the massage.*

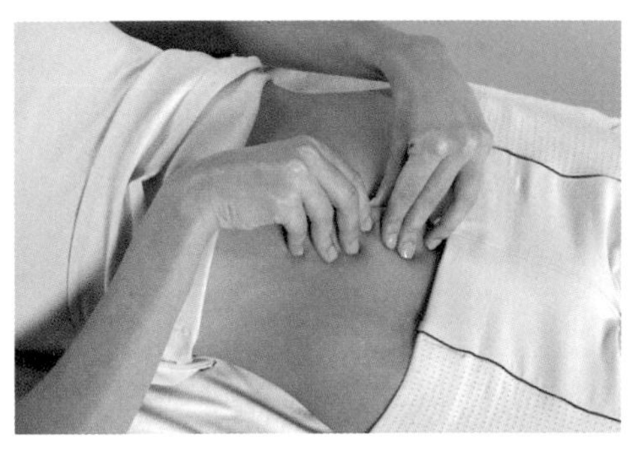

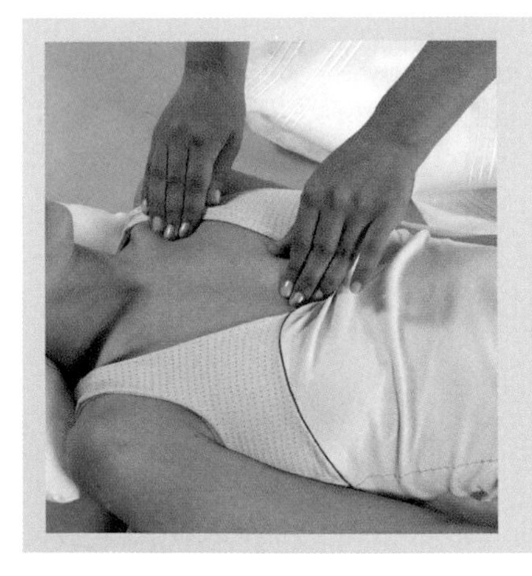

MASSAGE TO RELIEVE ANXIETY

To fight against negative emotional states that tend to appear before or during menstruation or during pregnancy and menopause, apply gentle finger pressure on the side of the sternum. This is where the points are found that release tension in the upper chest and the solar plexus (the seat of the emotions). It is best that a partner applies for it to be most effective.

Purifying and protecting massages

Lymphatic draining massage is mainly made up of slow, circular movements applied to the lymphatic circulatory system. This technique helps to eliminate toxins from the body and increase the immune system to protect the organism from disease.

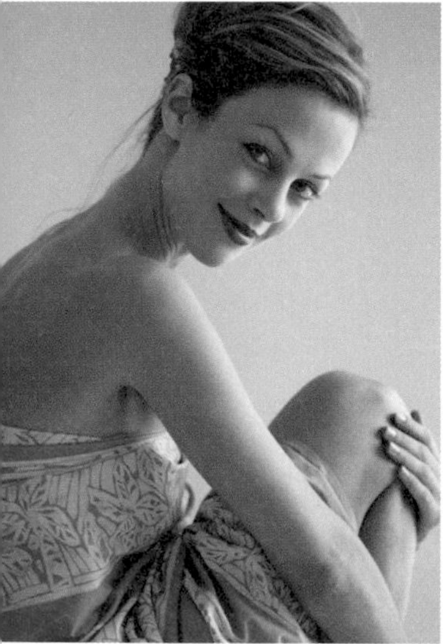

✚ Lymph is a clear fluid that circulates around the body tissues. The lymphatic system consists of thin tubes that run throughout the body. These tubes are called lymph vessels. The tubes branch through all parts of the body like the arteries and veins that carry blood. The fluid, called lymph, flows through the lymphatic system to the biggest lymph vessel –the thoracic duct. The thoracic duct then empties back into the blood circulation.

As the blood circulates, fluid leaks out into the body tissues. This fluid is important because it carries food to the cells and waste products back to the bloodstream. The leaked fluid drains into the lymph vessels. The lymphatic system helps fight infection in many ways, making the function of the lymphatic system part of the immune system. Lymphatic massage is supposed to strengthen the performance of the immune system, cleaning and draining toxins from the lymph system. The lymphatic vessels are irrigated, stimulating the lymph movement and the flow of nutrients and oxygen in the area. This massage might be beneficial during PMS because along with the retention of liquids in the body, excess toxins are also accumulated, causing your ankles to swell, headaches and other discomforts. This massage is also recommended during post-menopause, because it promotes rejuvenation and weight loss. Lymphatic drainage facilitates relaxation and lowering of stress, it also acts favorably against cellulitis.

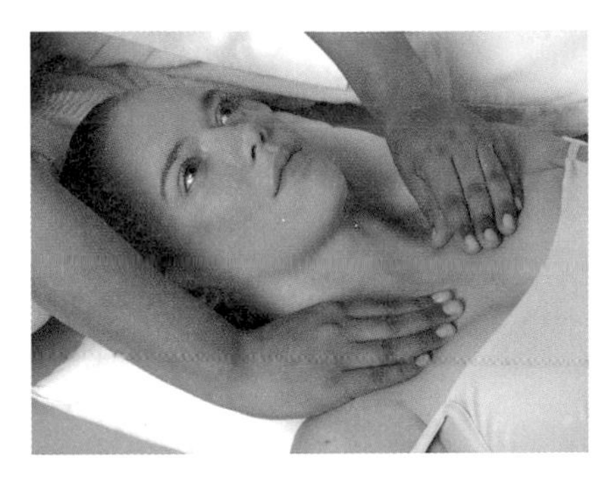

1. Begin by purifying the high chest area. Apply pressure with your fingertips and press 5 times, as if you were "pumping."

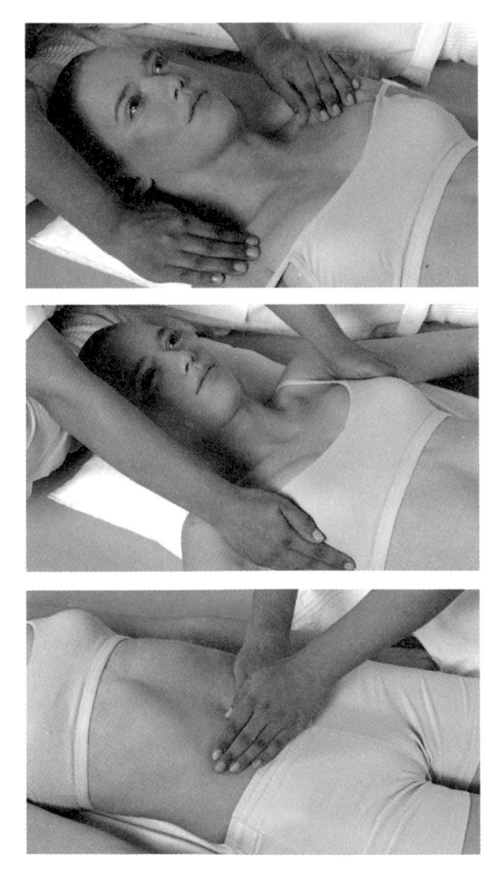

2. Slide the palms of your hands to the area of the neck, making series of odd movements 3, 5, or 7. This massage opens the vessels to the lymph system.

3. Massage the armpits with the fingers stretched out. You can use three or four of your fingers.

4. Continue to massage the abdomen, placing one hand on top of the other. This will help to purify the intestinal system.

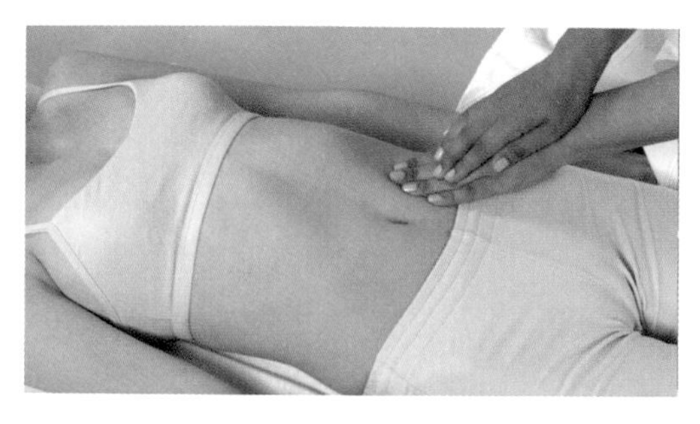

5. Continue to massage down the abdomen. Start on the left side, from the top, downward. The hands one on top of the other, applying gentle pressure.

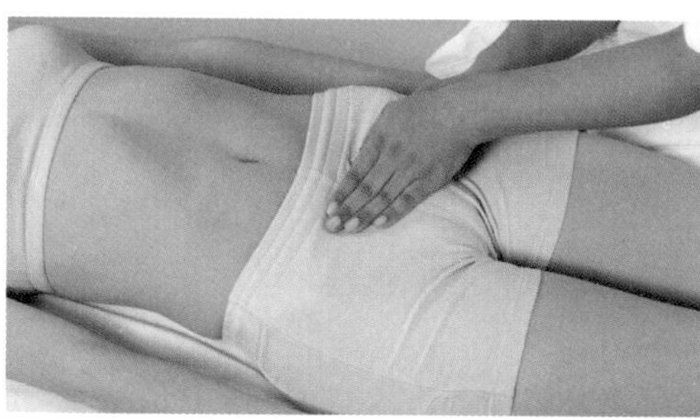

6. On the area below the abdomen, massage with your fingers stretched out and pushing toward the center. This helps to prevent varicose veins and fight cellulitis.

7. Massage from the knee to the pelvis, pressing and releasing (pumping motion) 3 to 5 times on the knee, the middle of the thigh and the pelvis.

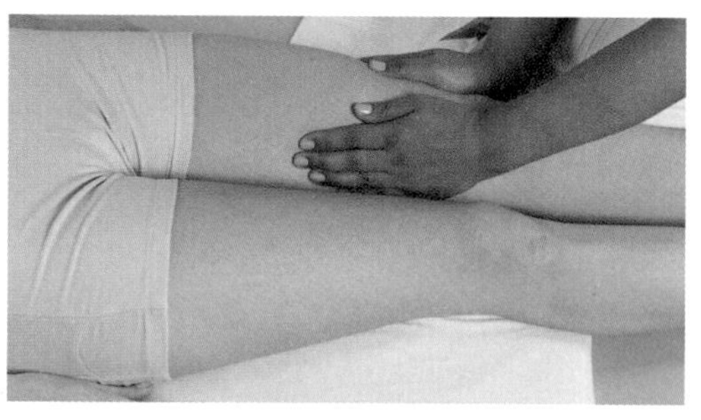

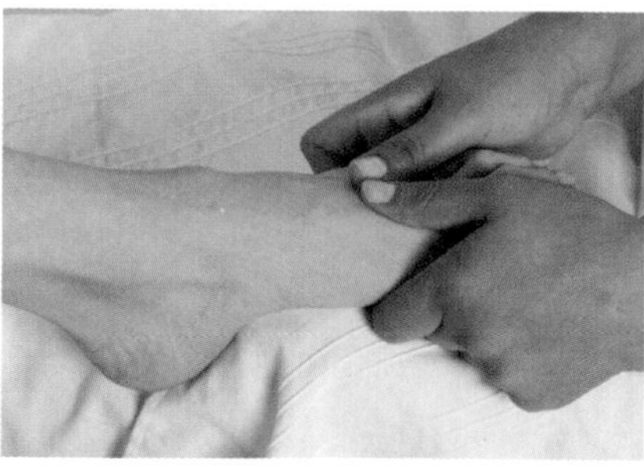

8. On the feet: on the top of the foot gently massage with the tips of your thumbs, in a circular motion.

OTHER RECOMMENDED MASSAGES

- **Quiromassage.** Employs a brushing, pumping and kneading technique for relaxation. Quiromassage reduces fatigue and releases tension built up in the back and abdomen.
- **Neuro-physiological massage.** Used to calm the nervous system, producing psychological relaxation, helping to fight stress.

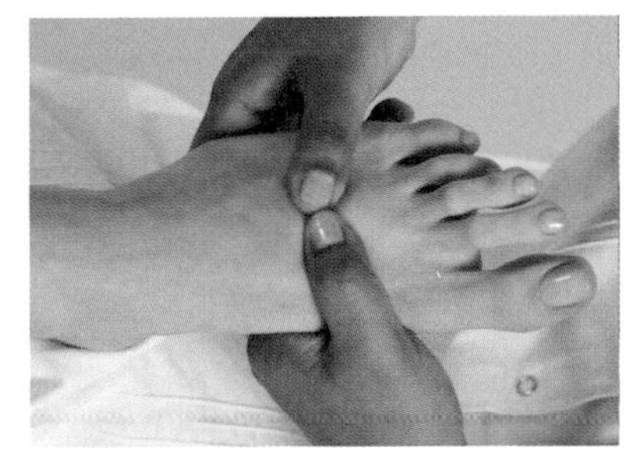

9. *Next, apply a ring of pressure on the top of the foot, as shown in the photo. This massage helps to reduce the accumulation of liquid that tends to build up in the area due to water retention.*

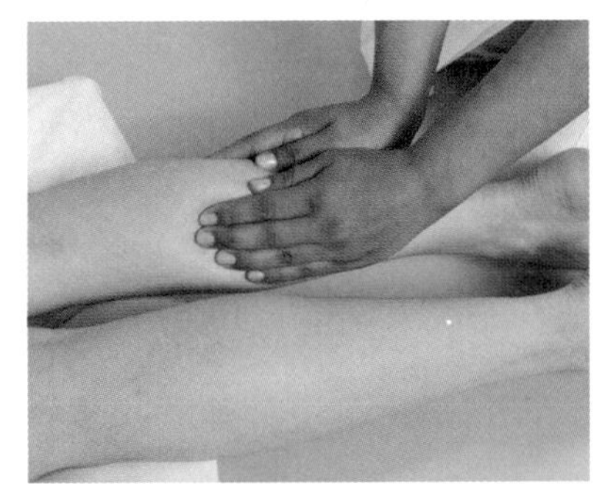

10. *Before the patient turns over, practice the previous series from below to the top. Once the patient turns over, start on the legs, applying gentle pressure with the palms of the hands on the calves.*

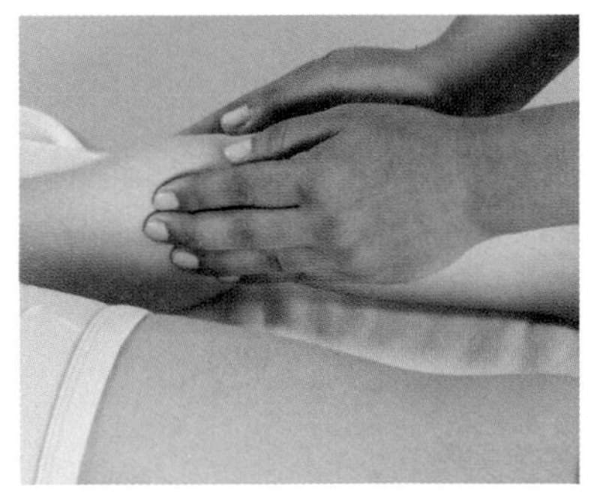

11. *Work on the arms, from the hands up to the shoulder. Purify the armpit by placing one hand over the other on the armpit. Apply pressure with your top hand.*

WARNING

Lymphatic drainage is not recommended for serious infections, heart problems, phlebitis, thrombosis, high blood pressure, skin infections, under active thyroid gland, bronchial asthma, cancer and symptoms of dizziness. This massage is recommended to treat PMS discomforts. It's best not to use this massage if you are suffering from irregular periods or during your period.

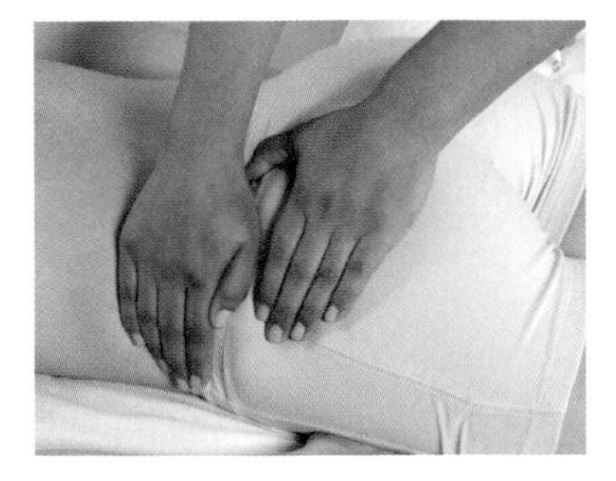

12. *Massage along the lower back with open hands. Before this step, it's recommended that you work on the sacrum area, so that the fluid in the buttocks flows to the pelvis.*

The power of water

Hydrotherapy is one of the most effective natural therapies to treat female discomforts. It helps you to relax and fight against the tension brought on by hormonal changes. The following is a guide to hydrotherapy techniques for each ailment.

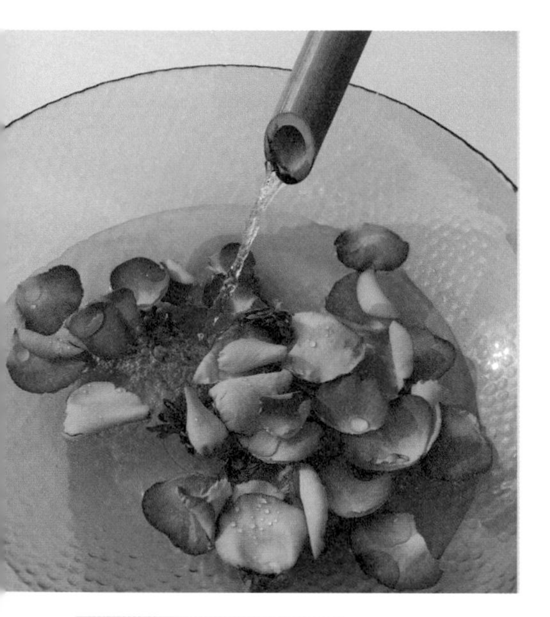

Water, in liquid, solid or vapor form, can be used as an effective therapy to treat typical female discomforts. Water helps to regulate the body's temperature, eliminate toxins and stimulate or calm the nervous system.

- A brief cold shower can help to energize you in cases of depression or anxiety.
- Applying warm or hot water over the entire

NOTE
You should always consult your physician before taking hydrotherapy practices.

RECOMMENDATIONS

- Hydrotherapy should be practiced in a warm, well-ventilated room.
- It's not recommended to practice this therapy right before or after eating meals.
- Do not hold your breath during treatment, you should keep breathing regulary.
- Before exposing the body to cold water, the body should be warmed up, and in a warm room. You should avoid using cold water therapy when your body is feeling weak; in this case it's advised to use hot baths that relax and lower your blood pressure.
- Always after using hydrotherapy, dry your face and your hair with a towel and leave the rest of the body moist, covering up with a blanket or comforter. After taking a baths, it's best to lie down in a warm, cozy bed.

body or specific parts of the body during a shower can help to soothe nervous tension brought on by PMS or menopause.

- Ice or cold water is very effective in reducing swelling in the ankles brought on by poor blood circulation or by water retention.
- Soaking in a hot bath helps to decongest and completely relax the body. However, women who suffer from low blood pressure should use caution.
- Steam baths, and other water treatments for female discomforts increase blood flow to the skin's surface, provoking sweating and at the same time cleaning the body from the inside out.
- Adding a few drops of essential oils to a vaporizer with hot steam, helps to bring on a deep sleep when you are having trouble sleeping, especially for pregnant women in the last trimester. (Essential oils recommended to bring on sleep are myrrh and tangerine, because they don't have any side effects.)
- Showers, especially if accompanied by a rubbing with a sponge or rough textured cloth, increase the skin's breathing and stimulate the metabolism, blood circulation and oxygen flow. This can be a key resource during menopause.
- Baths stimulate the irrigation of the abdominal and pelvic region, relieving premenstrual and menopause symptoms.

WATER EXERCISE

Recommended for menopause, pregnancy and PMS. You can use this therapy in the bathtub of your own home. It's refreshing, improves blood circulation, regulates the body's temperature, calms the nervous system and strengthens the veins in the legs. It can also be used to help bring on repairing sleep.

Instructions

- Fill the bathtub with cold water.
- Imitate a stork, (stand in the tub, kicking up water with each step) walk in the water for thirty seconds to one minute.
- Get out of the bathtub. Dry your body with your hands, not a towel.
- Put on cotton socks and walk around a warm room, until your legs warm up, or cover up in your bed.

Warning. This exercise is not recommended for women suffering from urinary tract infections, poor circulation or cramps in the legs.

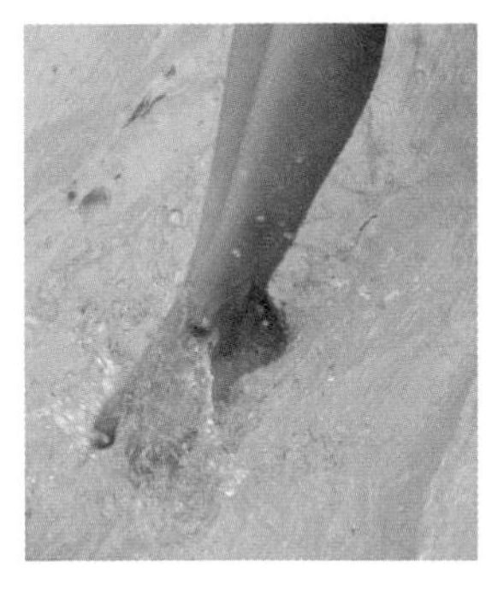

IMMEDIATE RELIEF

The following exercises are effective and easy for specific discomforts.

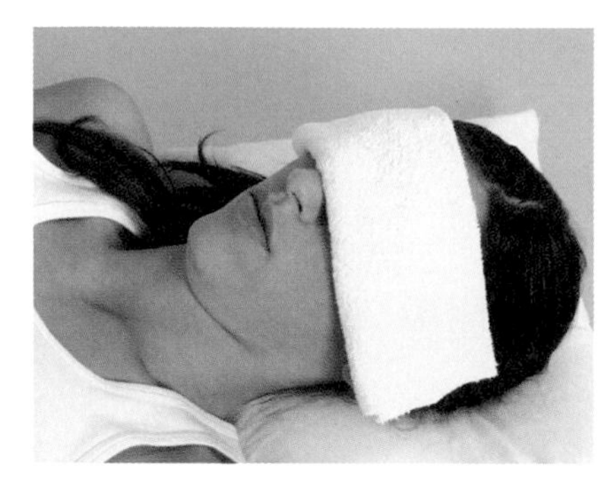

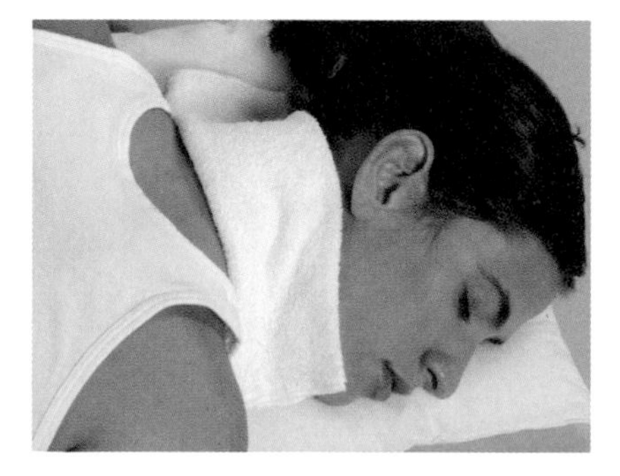

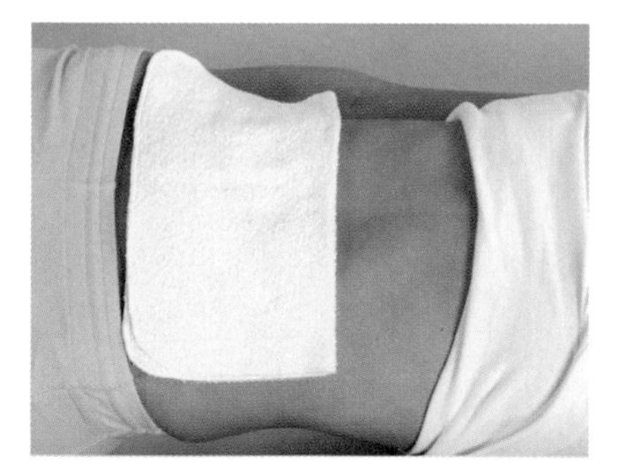

Bandages or clothes

Using bandages or linen cloths on specific points of the body, can help to relieve specific pains. They can be soaked in cold, tepid or hot water, depending on your discomfort. Wring the cloth out before placing it on your skin.

- **For headaches.** Water acts on symptoms related to headaches caused by premenstrual tension. For immediate relief, soak a linen cloth in cold water, wring it out and place it on your forehead or over your eyes. Rest with your eyes closed for as long as you feel comfortable. Continue to soak the cloth as many times as necessary.
- **For tension in the neck.** Alternating with cold and hot compresses on the back can help to relieve accumulated tension in this part of the body.
- **For abdominal pain.** Tepid compresses on the skin above the abdomen can bring a pleasant sense of warmth to relax the abdominal organs.

Effusions

Consists of applying spurts of varying temperatures of water on a specific point of the body, to relieve specific pains.

■ **For uterus pains during PMS.**
It's recommended an effusion on the abdominal region. Using a hand held showerhead apply warm water on the muscles, and continue upward at the base of the rib cage. This is not only helpful for uterus pains, but also helps to relax the entire body and to improve the metabolism and digestion. Apply water for three or four minutes, using the showerhead to release constant and strong water pressure.

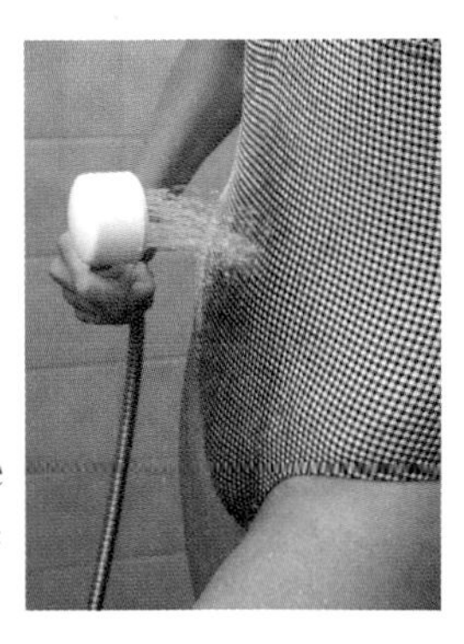

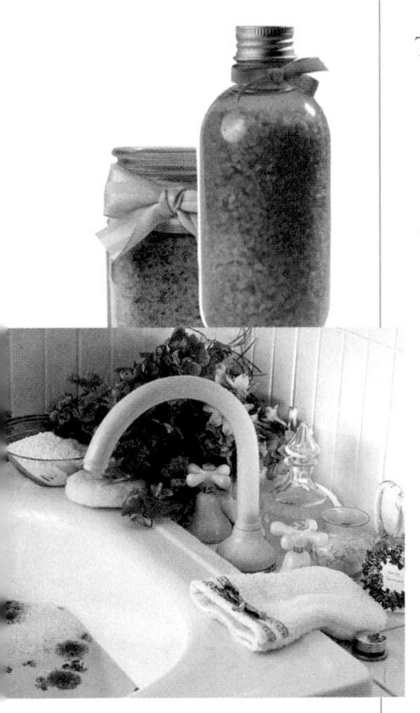

HEALING BATHS

There's nothing more comforting than drawing a warm bath (hot but not too hot) and adding a few drops of essential oils to relieve particular symptoms. Imagine soaking away the pain.

- ***For circulatory problems***

Add 2 cups of sea salt or 3-4 drops of cyprus and/or camomile essential oils to a bathtub filled with hot water. Soak for 10 minutes to improve circulatory problems caused by PMS.

- ***To fight water retention.***

Hormonal activity before menstruation and during your period tends to cause water retention, causing your ankles to swell and straining your kidneys and liver. To help fight symptoms draw a hot bath with a mixed herbal infusion. You can add essential oils of orange, camomile or rose.

- ***For your skin during pregnancy.***

During pregnancy women tend to suffer from skin irritation. To prevent your skin from reacting take a warm bath, with equal quantities of oatmeal and lime buds in a linen cloth bag soaked in the water. As an alternative you can soften the skin by adding a cloth bag with chopped cucumber. If your skin is continuously irritated, soak a cotton ball in spring water and apply on the affected areas after the bath. ***Safety.*** *Pregnant women should avoid sauna baths, Turkish baths and soaking in hot water.*

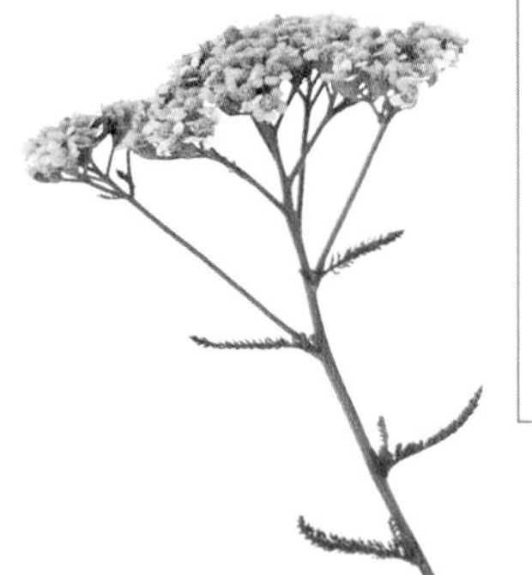

More alternatives

Many female discomforts affect women's emotions. Colors, crystals, art and laughing can work as natural therapies to lift up the spirits and fight against the symptoms.

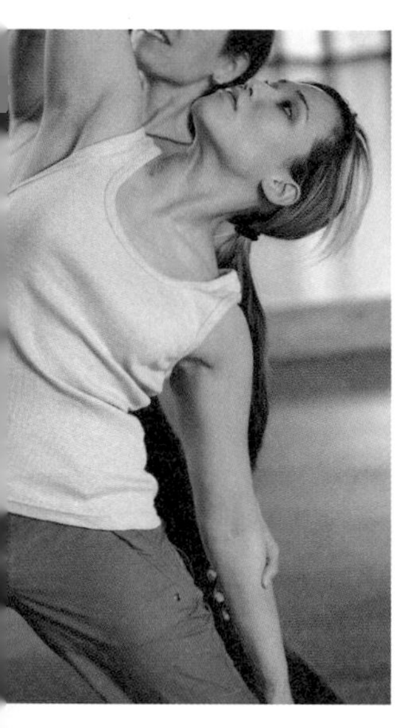

✚ Incorporating color, music and art into your life is not a minor task. All of these therapies, along with crystal therapy carry vibrations that lift up your spirits and give you a better outlook on life. Many complementary therapies use these resources for improving overall well-being.

HEALING ART

Art therapy is a way of healing that may benefit the nervous system, balance hormones and stimulate neurological brain signals. This is why art, in whatever form, can help to relieve the aches and pains suffered by women. Art may help to connect you to your psyche, where you store your creative powers. Through artistic expression, you may experience a change of attitude, emotional state or sense of pain, which helps you to relax and release your body and imagination. It's not important to be artistic; this therapy encourages women to let their creative capacities flow to aid a true curing process that can be expressed through painting, dancing, sculpture, literary expression or any other creative expression.

SOFT MUSIC

This type of music affects the right side of the brain, related to our emotional activity. Listening to New Age. classical or baroque music helps prevent stressful or negative thoughts. Blood pressure, cardiac rhythum, breathing and muscular tension diminish when endorfins and serotonin are released, giving an overall sense of well-being.

The arts that are considered the most appropriate for lifting up your spirits, improving the function of the immune system and the proper functioning of the body include:

■ **Music.** Music has a positive effect on the body. Studies have shown that when humans listen to music they release endorphins, a biochemical compound naturally produced in our bodies that is more potent than morphine in fighting pain. Soft melodies help your body to relax, improves your humor and give you motivation, helping you to fight against the depressive symptoms sometimes brought on by feminine discomforts. Among other positive physical effects, musics influences your breathing, blood pressure, stomach cramps and your hormone levels. Your heart rhythm either speeds up or slows down, depending on the musical rhythm. Music can also influence the electric rhythms in the brain.

■ **Dancing.** Dance therapy can help to improve body image and self-confidence, reducing fear and physical tension. Through dance you can release your emotions and help to reduce chronic pain. Dancing not only releases endorphins but also combines with the powerful effects of music, that promote healthy interpersonal relationships, helping to keep you in high spirits and in a good mood.

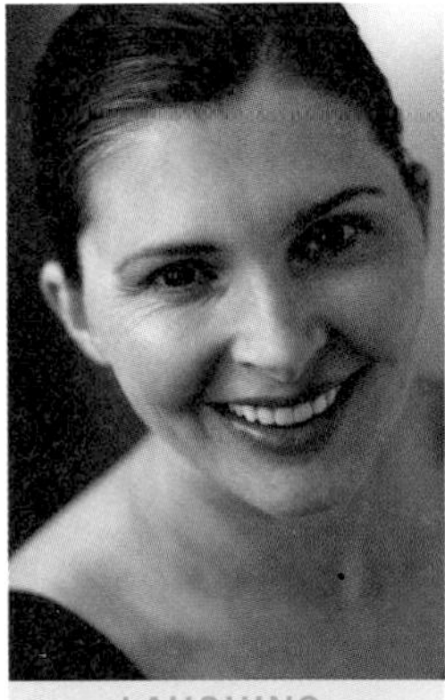

LAUGHING, A SERIOUS THERAPY

Sigmund Freud attributed laughter as an aid in helping to improve mental health and in releasing negative energy. Recent studies have shown that laughter releases endorphins, the body's natural painkiller, and so is a pleasant act, producing a general feeling of well-being. However, more than this, laughter has been shown to considerably benefit one's health and even battle disease. Laughter is a great way to eliminate negative emotional, physical, mental and sexual blocks.

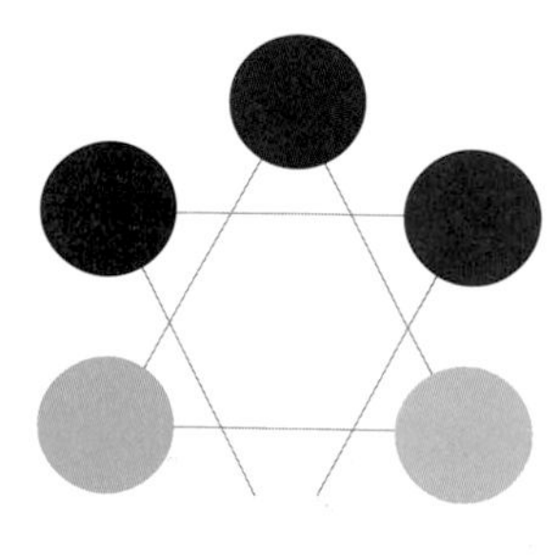

APPLICATION OF CHROMOTHERAPY
This simple and efficient system consists of using a chromotherapy lamp or light bulb (between 60 and 100 watts), covering the lamp post with the transparent pure colors needed, or combined colors. Varying different transparencies you can follow sequences or quick changes of color from the light emitted, depending on what treatment is recommended.

COLOR IS LIFE

Color therapy is a set of principles used to create harmonious color for healing. According to the principles of this therapy, color is energy. It is a form of energy medicine based on the belief that the human body is composed of energy fields. Color therapy stimulates different centers of the brain and works on problems related to energy deficiencies that cause a number of physical and psychological responses in the body. Some alternatives for using colors include:

- **In rooms and in your home.** Paint interior walls inside your home or your office the color appropriate for the problem you are suffering. You can also use color panels.
- **On your body.** Wear clothes or accessories the color appropriate for each discomfort.
- **Direct therapeutic application.** Filtered lamps that reflect different tones. Objects or adornments with stones or colored crystals.

The most appropriate colors to treat female discomforts include the following:

- **Red.** Gives off stimulating energy which is why it is recommended during your period or the menopause when you feel low on energy.
- **Yellow.** It's recommended when you are having a difficult feminine day. This color radiates well-being, happiness, confidence and improves your self-esteem. It is effective when you are going through emotional instability, facing fears or suffering from headaches. Yellow foods give off light and may help to fight depression.
- **Green.** This is an excellent detoxifying color. It helps to regenerate your body's cells

and relaxes the muscles. Stimulates creativity and releases tension.

■ **Blue.** For its relaxing and sedative effects, it's ideal for women who suffer from insomnia or have trouble sleeping soundly, especially during pregnancy.

■ **Violet.** Acts as a purifier of the body, helping to remove toxins. It's recommended to use violet when you are menstruating.

GEM ENERGY

According to gemtherapy, semiprecious stones, through their energy and vibrations are excellent treatments for improving physical and mental health. The following gems are the most widely used to treat female discomforts.

■ **Pearls.** Related to feminine energy, they are good to use during pregnancy. Also, pearls have a calming effect that helps to sooth irritability and anger brought on by PMS.

■ **Topaz.** Improves circulation, allowing greater oxygen flow to the brain. It's recommended during menopause. Related to hope, optimism and faith in a good future.

■ **Emerald.** This gem is recommended for menopause for its beneficial effects on the skeleton and bones.

■ **Sapphire.** Appropriate for treating bouts of depression, because it is said to absorb the negative energy that generates sadness. Sapphire's vibrations are also useful for treating nervous problems.

■ **Cornelian.** This stone represents happiness. It increases energy and transmits well-being to whoever wears it.

■ **Garnet.** This stone is recommended during menstruation, because it is said to regulate blood circulation and relieve aches and pains.

HOW TO USE GEMS

After practicing a relaxation session, find the stone or stones recommended for your discomfort and place them around you, preferably on the skin (with adhesive tape). Wash the stone with salted water every day and expose it to sunlight in a glass of mineral water. Drinking this water may also be beneficial.

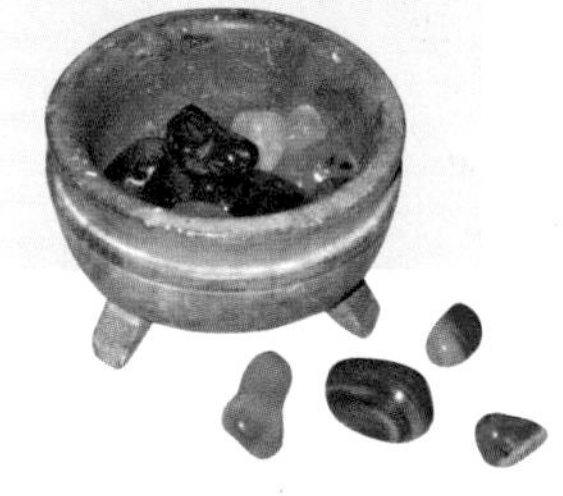

Nature's way of taking care of a woman

Many medicinal plants can make up effective remedies to relieve female discomforts. Essential oils made from herbs and flowers, mentioned in *Essential Oils from A to Z* box, are used topically, according to aromatherapy recommendations, and help the overall well-being of women.

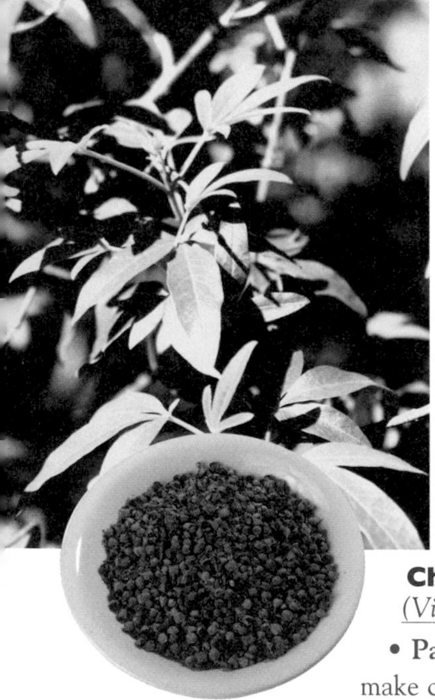

Nothing is better than natural remedies to relieve symptoms that are also, on the whole, natural such as most female discomforts. Many medicinal herbs provide a gentle remedy without side effects. The following are effective medical plants and herbal remedies to fight back pains and ailments. Some plants may be easier to find than others depending on where the plants are cultivated. You can find some as fresh plants or dried, and others in liquid form, tinctures, tablets or powder.

Chasteberry
(Vitex agnus castus)

- **Parts used.** The fruit, which is used to make capsules and extracts.
- This tree grows in the Mediterranean countries and Central Asia. The dried fruits, which has a pepper-like aroma and flavor, is used.
- Chasteberry could be considered a women's herb. It has the effect of stimulating and normalizing pituitary gland functions, especially its progesterone function. The greatest use of chasteberry lies in normalizing

NOTE
You should always consult your physician before starting any herbal treatment.

AROMATHERAPY

Is a system which treats different ailments via the use of essential oils extracted from plants, flowers, trees and shrubs. These are highly potent and concentrated extracts which are mixed with a vegetable oil, that acts as a carrier of each essence. Essential oils are applied to skin through massage or via drops added to the bath, –they can also be inhaled with a vaporizer– always under medical supervision. When used in baths and massages they center the system by penetrating the skin and the sense of smell. To know which are the most appropriate essences for relieving female discomforts see Essential Oils from A to Z *box.*

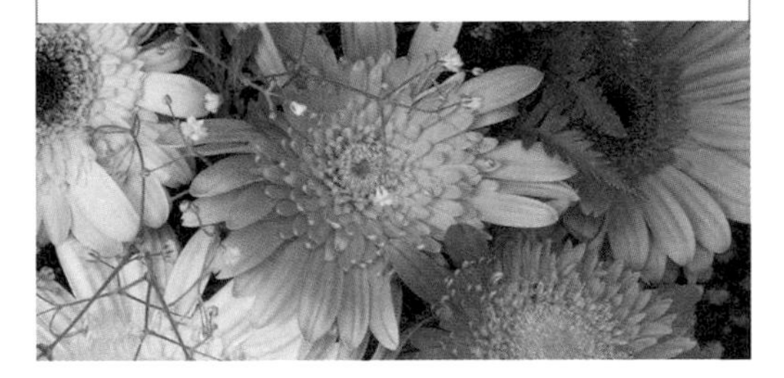

the activity of the female sex hormones, it is thus indicated for premenstrual stress and other disorders related to hormone function such as migraines, acne during puberty, menopause and infertility.

• **Warning.** Chasteberry is not recommended for use during pregnancy or while breast-feeding. If taken in excess it can be toxic.

PREMENSTRUAL SYNDROME

To help relieve aches and discomforts related to your periods you can take capsules or extract of chasteberry for four months, until your symptoms subside. To find out what is the appropriate dose, you should consult your doctor.

ESSENTIAL OILS FROM A TO Z

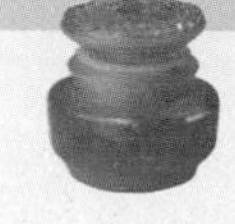

CYPRUS

Has a regulating effect on the female reproductive system, relieving menstrual discomforts. It also stimulates blood circulation and regulates excess heat and fluids in the body. Blends with juniper, lavender, lemon, rosemary and marjoram.

Safety. It shouldn't be used during pregnancy. During massages it's recommended to use without applying pressure to varicose veins.

EUCALYPTUS

Its clean, potent and refreshing aroma strengthens the nervous system and has a stimulating effect. Recommended for treating the negative emotions common with PMS and menopause. Blends well with juniper, lemon, lemon herb, lemon balm and rosemary.

Safety. Shouldn't be used in cases of high blood pressure or epilepsy. Use in low doses to prevent skin irritation.

WARNING

Essential oils are for external use **only**, they should **never** be ingested. Keep stored away from children and keep away from your eyes.

Angelica

(Angelica sinensis)

- **Parts used.** Roots, hips of the root, leaves, stems and seeds are used to make capsules and tinctures or in infusions.
- There are three variants of angelica: European, American and Chinese. The Chinese species is recommended to treat female discomforts.
- This herb may be very useful for painful or irregular menstrual periods, or as a tonic during menopause to improve circulation for cold hands and feet.
- **Warning.** Angelica should not be used during pregnancy.

Shepherd's purse

(Capsella bursa pastoris)

- **Parts used.** The entire plant, especially the stem. It is commercially cultivated to dry for making infusions.
- This plant belongs to the crucifer family. It gets its particular name from its fruits, it looks like the bag shepherds carry in some regions.
- It's principal use is to regulate menstrual flow, in cases of excessive menstruation and when your menstrual flow is little or irregular; it is an effective tonic for the uterus. Because of its anti-hemorrhage properties it is used for nosebleeds.

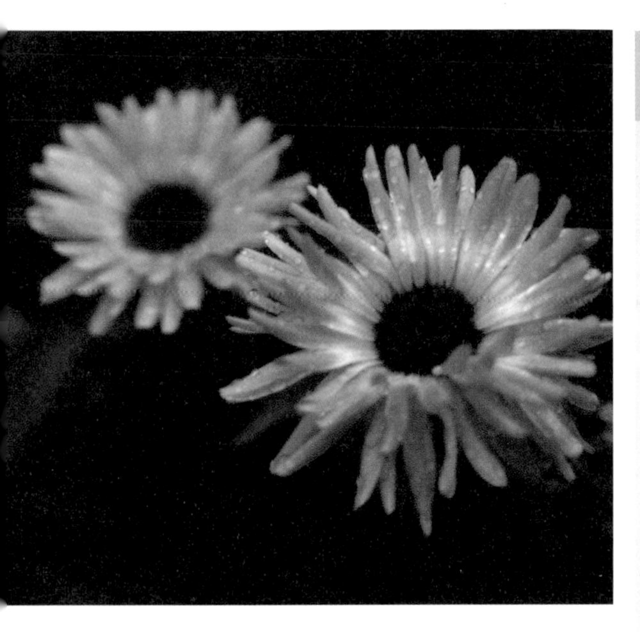

Marigold

(Calendula officinalis)

- **Parts used.** Flowers and leaves, for infusions.
- Native to Europe, this plant is grown in gardens. It looks like a daisy, but with yellow or orange petals.
- The plant can be used internally for the reproductive system, because it relieves menstrual problems, regulating the cycle. Because of its antiseptic, antibacterial and fungicidal properties, it's recommended to treat candidiasis.

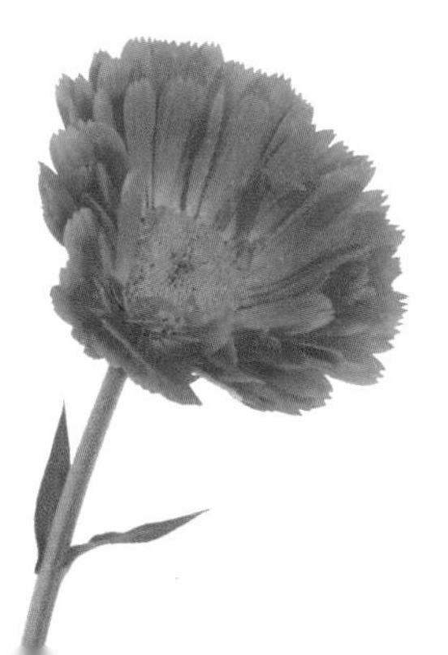

FOR SWELLING OR ACHY BREASTS

Prepare an infusion with marigold flowers and apply a compress soaked in this infusion to the sore area.

ESSENTIAL OILS FROM A TO Z

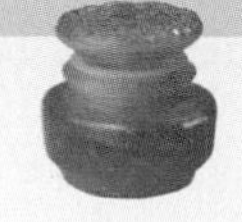

FENNEL

Aromatic and spicy aroma, similar to aniseed, increases the energy and self-esteem. Because of its estrogen content, it's good for relieving menstrual pains and PMS symptoms. It's also used to relieve symptoms of nausea and vomiting. Blends with geranium, lavender, lemon, rosemary, basil and sandalwood.

Safety. Shouldn't be used during pregnancy and for those who suffer from epilepsy, or for small children.

GERANIUM

This is a tonic for the circulatory system, appropriate for treating PMS. Relieves headaches, tones the nervous system and fights depression, reducing stress and nervous tension. Blends with Angelica, bergamot, grapefruit, lime, neroli and patchouli.

Safety. In high doses geranium can irritate the skin.

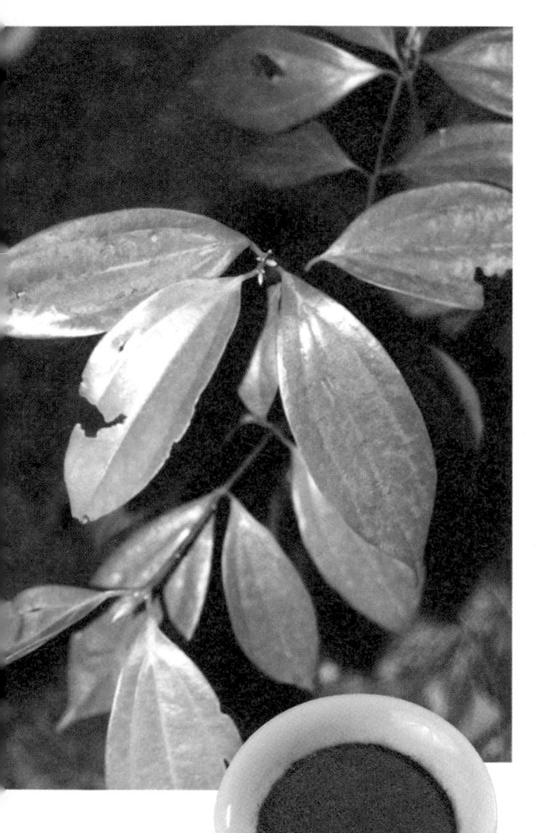

Cinnamon

(Cinnamomum verum sin.)

• **Parts used.** The inner bark of young tree branches.

• It's cultivated in Southeast Asia, in India, Madagascar and other tropical regions in South America.

• It's normally used for its digestive properties, helps to relieve nausea and vomiting, making it recommended during pregnancy. It also helps to improve the appetite and improves digestion in general.

• **Warning.** Not recommended for those who suffer from peptic gastric duodenal ulcers.

TO FIGHT NAUSEA

Prepare an infusion with 1 or 2 sticks of cinnamon per cup of water. You can add lemon slices. Drink 1 cup after meals. Keep in mind that it's more effective if drunk unsweetened.

Milk Thistle

(Carduus marianus)

• **Parts used.** Seeds and leaves.

• This stout, annual or biennial plant is found in dry, rocky soils in Southern and Western Europe and in some parts of the US.

INFUSION FOR BREAST-FEEDING
Crush or grind the seeds. Use 1 small teaspoon of crushed seeds per cup of boiling water. Allow to steep for a few minutes and drink before meals.

- An excellent remedy to increase the production of breast milk. Recommended for people who suffer from low blood pressure, to prevent sudden drops in pressure.
- **Warning.** Not recommended for those who suffer from high blood pressure.

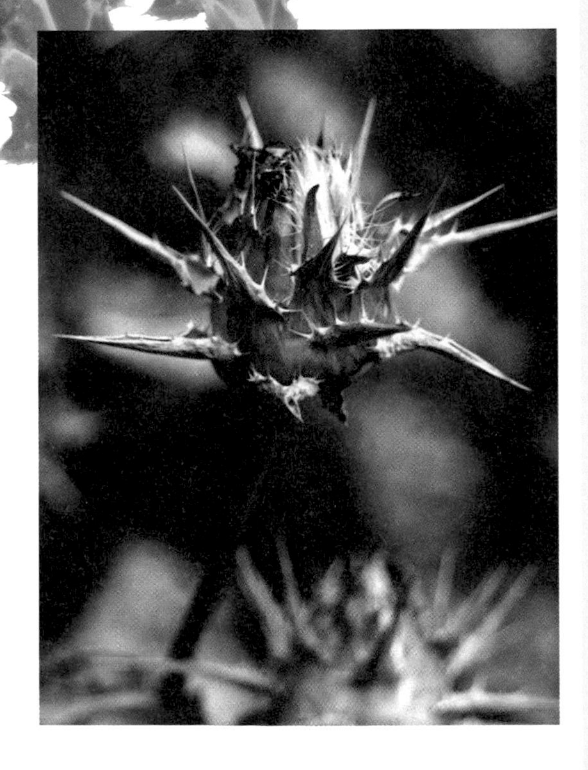

ESSENTIAL OILS FROM A TO Z

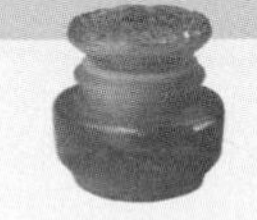

JASMINE

Works as a hormonal regulator, effective against postpartum depression. Relieves menstrual pain and vaginal infections, in addition to calming the nerves and lifting up spirits. Blend with myrrh, geranium, lime, neroli, rose, ylang ylang and sandalwood.

Safety. Should not be used during pregnancy, only to relieve childbirth pains.

JUNIPER

Clears, stimulates and tones the mind, lifting the spirits in moments of anxiety. Relieves cystitis, regulates the menstrual cycle and calms pains during menstruation. Blends well with clary sage, cypress, myrrh, grapefruit, and sandalwood.

Safety. Shouldn't be used during pregnancy, because it might induce labor. Should be used in low doses to protect the skin against irritation.

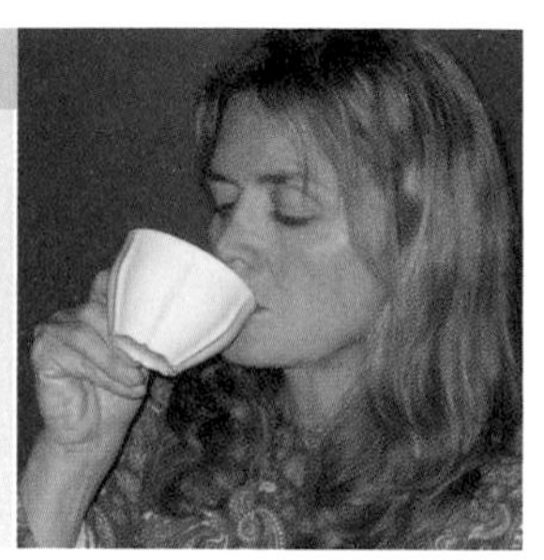

HORMONAL REGULATOR

Prepare an infusion with black cohosh root, chaste berry, wild yam, ginseng, liquorice and fennel. Drink 3 times a day during the second half of the menstrual cycle, for at least 3 months, to help regulate hormone levels.

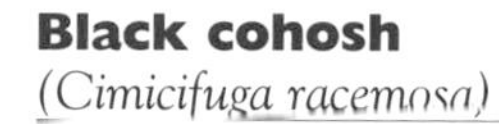

Black cohosh

(Cimicifuga racemosa)

- **Parts used.** Roots and root heads.
- Native to Canada, United States and Europe. It gets its name from the root, a black color.
- Used to relieve female discomforts such as pains and menstrual cramps, lack of estrogen or excess progesterone, high blood pressure and symptoms of menopause such as hot flashes and depression.
- **Warning.** Do not take during pregnancy or breastfeeding, or if you suffer from low blood pressure.

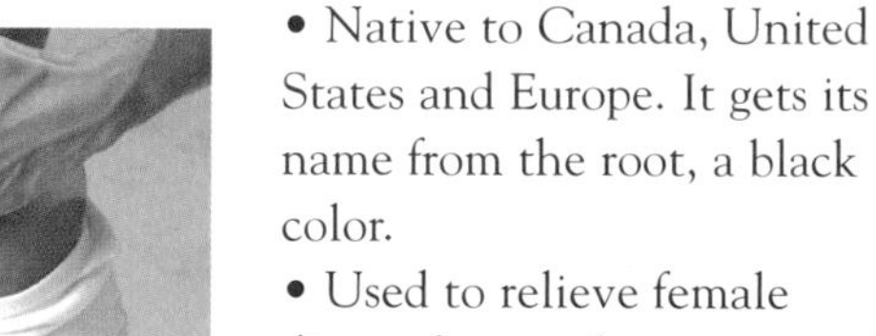

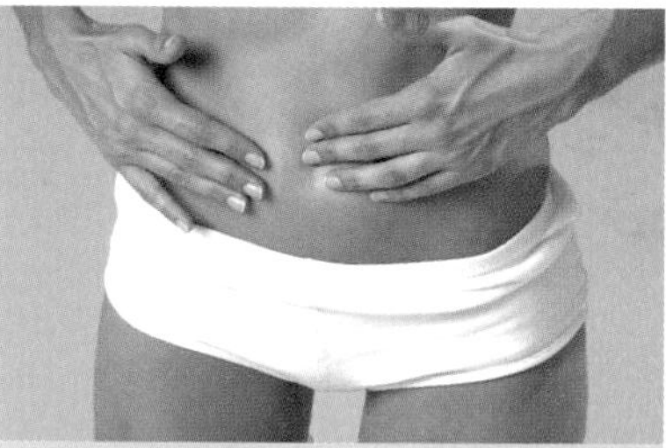

ANTI-SPASMODIC DECOCTION

Place 1 teaspoon of black cohosh powder in 3 cups of water and boil. Cool and drain.

Warning. Do not drink more than 1/2 cup, 2 times a day.

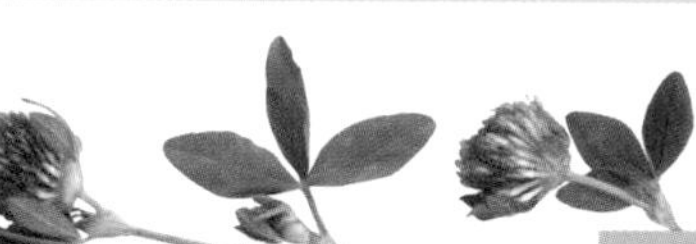

RED CLOVER FOR HOT FLASHES

Red clovers are rich in isoflavone compounds, between 10 and 20 times higher than soy. This herb may help to reduce the frequency and intensity of hot flashes and nocturnal sweating. It's advised to use it in low doses.

Dill

(Anethum graveolens)

• **Parts used**. The seeds and leaves are used in infusions and to make essential oils.

• Its properties have been understood for millenia, its use is mentioned in Egyptian papyrus and later in the Greek and Roman cultures.

• Coumarins, flavonoids, phenolic acids and chlorogene are the active compounds in dill for nursing mothers, to promote the flow of milk. It can also be used as a mild diuretic, and for light cases of bruising, water retention and small changes in blood pressure.

FEMININE INFUSION

Place 1 teaspoonful of dried dill root for every cup of boiling water and sit to steep; filter and drink. It should be taken after meals.

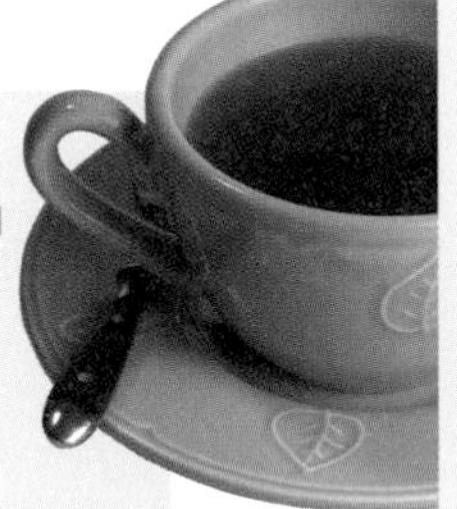

ESSENTIAL OILS FROM A TO Z

LAVENDER

Relieves mood swings brought on by PMS and menopause, at the same time having a regulating effect on the central nervous system and helping you sleep better. It is also effective in cases of depression or anger. Used with marjoram it calms menstrual pains. Blend with geranium, jasmine, lemon, camomile, rose and pine.

Safety. Do not use during pregnancy.

LEMON

Recommended during menopause for its toning effects on the nervous and circulatory systems. It helps to get rid of dead skin cells, lowers blood pressure and strengthens the immune system. Blend with eucalyptus, lavender, camomile and rose.

Safety. Use in low doses to avoid skin irritation. It's not recommended exposing your skin to direct sunlight after applying lemon to the skin.

RESTORE NATURALLY WITH NETTLES

Nettles are an excellent remedy to help you recover during menopause. They can be added to soups and stews, or use them as spinach to prepare a sauce to accompany pastas.

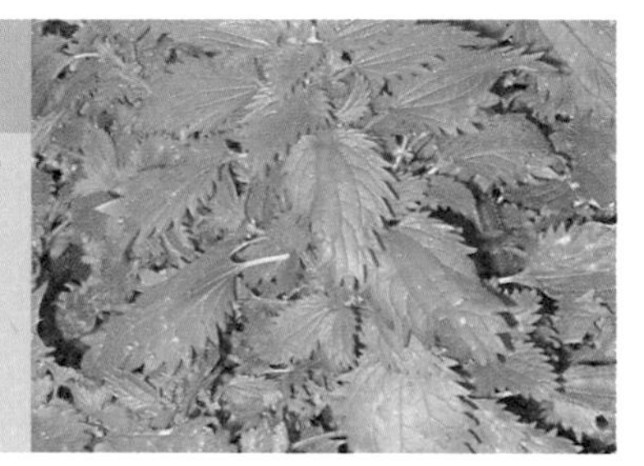

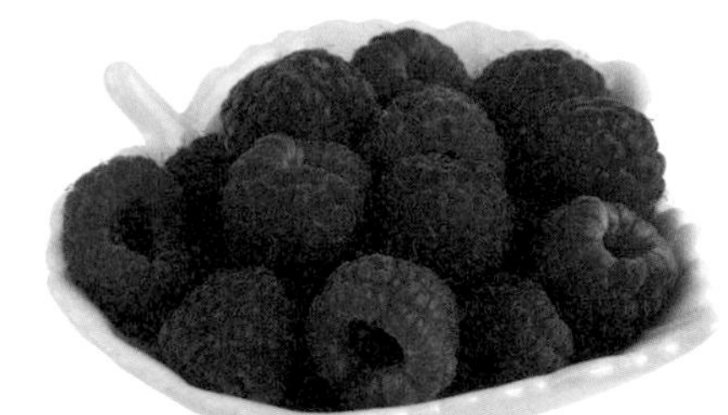

NATURAL DIURETIC. **Add 1/2 teaspoon of raspberry leaves to 1 cup of water, previously boiled. Let the leaves steep in the water, off the stove for 12 minutes. Drain and drink. As a diuretic, you can drink up to 3 cups a day. It's recommended for cases of oliguria, nephrolithiasis and cystitis**

Raspberry

(Rubus idaeus)

- **Parts used.** The leaves and flowers.
- Raspberry bushes grow mostly in mountainous regions.
- Raspberry is used as a diuretic, laxative and anti-inflammatory. One of its most important uses is against feminine and menstrual pains. It is very useful against water retention and swelling. In addition, it is high in vitamin C.

Fennel

(Foeniculum vulgare)

- **Parts used.** Roots, seeds and leaves are used to make infusion and decoctions, they are also used to make an essence, which can be ingested. But the essential oil is only for topical use.
- Fennel is a biennial or perennial plant that grows wild in the Mediterranean area and in Asia Minor, but is commonly cultivated in the US and Europe.
- The essence is extracted from the leaves and is an excellent remedy for colic and for breast-feeding mothers. Fennel has been used to promote menstruation in women. It may be useful to relieve the pains of menopause in older women.

• Used externally, fennel has anti-inflammatory properties, effective in fighting pain. The root is a diuretic (helping to drain liquids) which is why it is used for cystitis.

• **Warning.** In high doses, taking the flowers can provoke convulsions. It's not recommended for epileptics. Do not use during pregnancy or for small children or newborns.

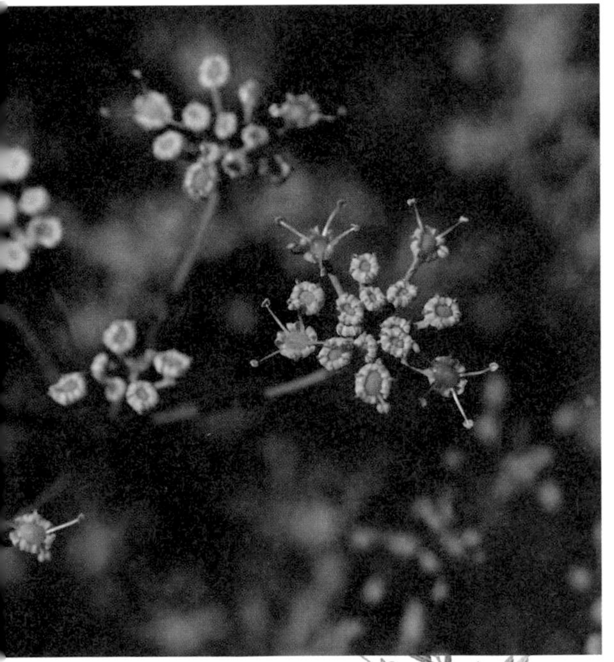

FRESH FENNEL CATAPLASM

Its mild estrogenic effect is partially responsible for the use of fennel for milk production. Use with a compress on the breasts to stimulate milk production.

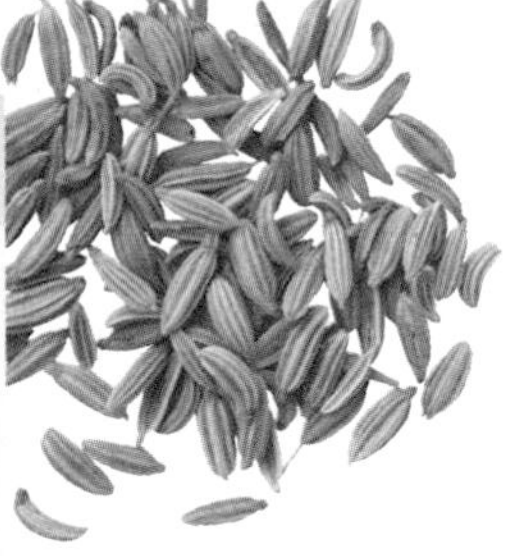

ESSENTIAL OILS FROM A TO Z

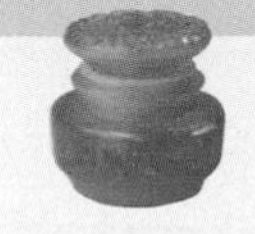

LEMON BALM

Regulates menstruation, relieves menstrual pains. It is a tonic for the uterus. Blend with myrrh, jasmine, juniper, rose, marjoram, ylang ylang.

Safety. Do not use during pregnancy. It can irritate sensitive skin.

MYRRH

Helps to relax the body with its warm, resonant and penetrating aroma. May be added to bath water during menstruation for its calming effects, it's recommended to use during childbirth. Blends with geranium, grapefruit, lime, neroli, sandalwood and vetiver.

SANDALWOOD

Stimulates the immune system and at the same time reduces nervous tension and anxiety brought on by PMS and menopause. Blends with myrrh, geranium, rose, vetiver.

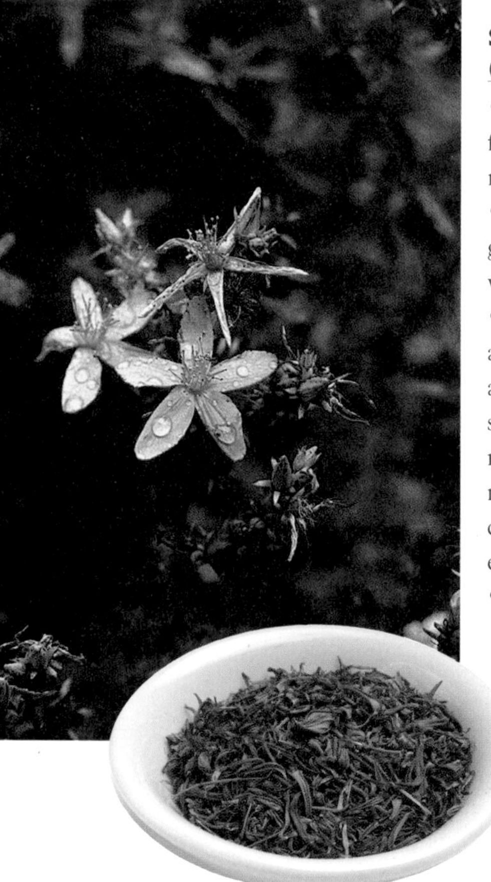

St. John's Wort

(Hypericum perforatum)

• **Parts used.** Leaves and flowers are used fresh or dry to make infusions.

• Native to Europe, today it is grown in many parts of the world.

• Calming agent against slight and moderate depression. Acts as a tonic for the nervous system and especially for the reproductive system during menopause and during physical changes that cause mental or emotional instability.

• **Warning.** Avoid exposure to direct sunlight if you are taking St. John's Wort for treatment, because it increases your skin's sensibility and can cause your skin to react with spots and inflammations.

Flax

(Linum usitatissimum)

• **Parts used.** The seeds, called "flax".

• Native to the Mediterranean but is cultivated in a number of countries in Europe and the American continent where the climate is moderate.

• For menstrual pain, apply a compress with flaxseed flour as an effective remedy, because of its antispasmodic, sedative and anti-inflammatory properties.

• The seeds, when ingested with abundant liquid can act as a gentle laxative, indicated for fighting the abdominal ailments that accompany menopause.

• **Warning.** The oil found in flaxseed flour makes the flour turn rancid rapidly, this can irritate the skin.

FLAX FOR MENOPAUSE

Due to its antioxidant, antiseptic and anti-tumor properties, it's recommended to eat bread or other foods with flaxseed added. Use flaxseed as a condiment in salads and soups. You can also dress salads using flaxseed oil.

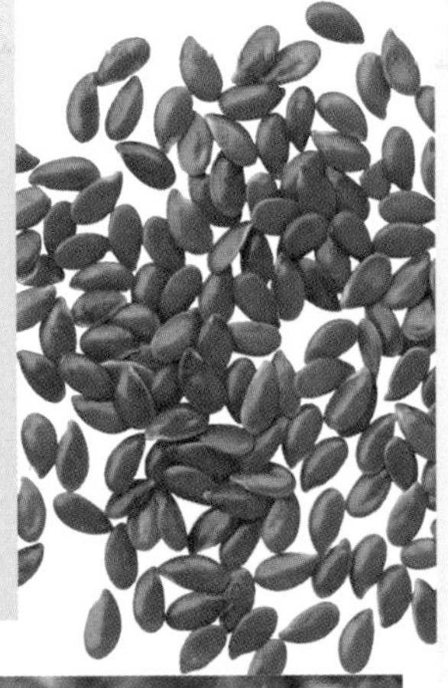

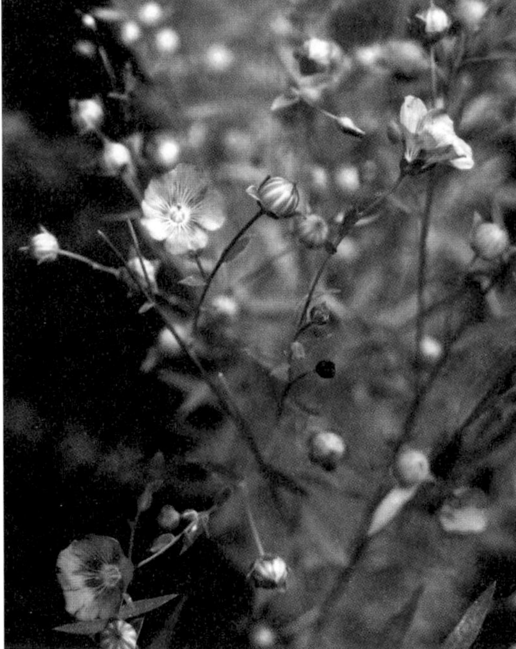

ESSENTIAL OILS FROM A TO Z

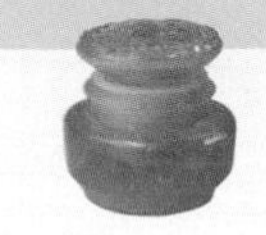

TANGERINE

This oil is very beneficial because it regulates the metabolic processes, water retention and cellulitis. It also might help to relieve PMS, reduce stretch marks on the skin and improve blood circulation to the skin's surface. Blends with grapefruit, lavender, neroli, basil and ylang ylang.

Safety. This oil makes your skin more sensitive to the sun. Avoid direct sunlight exposure after using on the skin.

TEA TREE

Its fresh and clean aroma helps to tone and restore, while fortifying the immune system. It also helps to relieve candidiasis.

It combines with eucalyptus, cypress, lavender, pine and ylang ylang.

Safety. It can be used pure as an antiseptic, but before hand you should test your skin for sensitivity and only apply to the affected area.

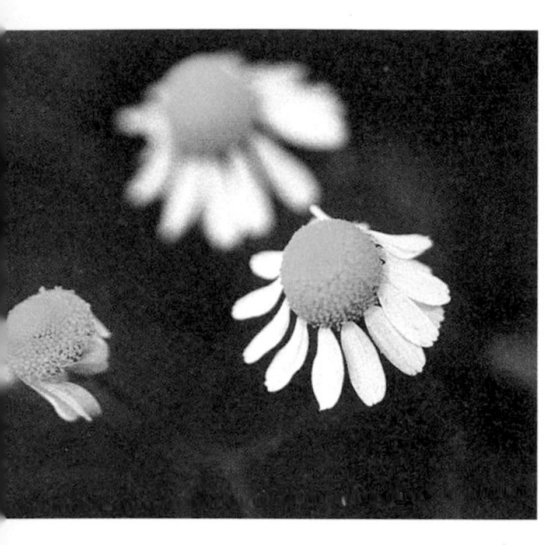

Camomile

(Chamomilla recutita)

• **Parts used.** The flowers to prepare infusions or to make essential oils.

• An effective sedative, helping to bring on sleep and relieve stress and tensions brought on by PMS and menopause. It is also recommended for cases of nausea, especially morning sickness during pregnancy, although only in infusions.

• **Warning.** Pregnant women should not use camomile essential oil during pregnancy, topically or internally. Some people can become sensitive or develop skin allergies in contact with this plant or taking infusions made with it.

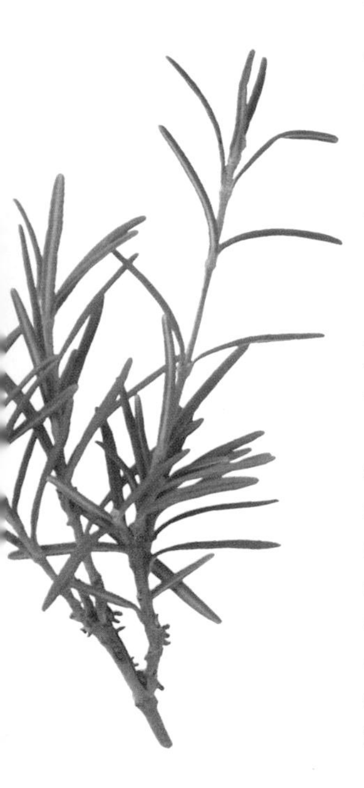

Rosemary

(Rosmarinus officinalis)

• **Parts used.** The leaves are used to prepare infusions or make essential oil.

• Native to the Mediterranean, this plant is known throughout the world for its culinary uses.

• Carries anti-inflammatory, antispasmodic, antioxidant and toning properties. It's recommended for menopause, because it helps to drain fluids to the brain, improving memory retention and concentration. It can also be used for depressive states and apathy. To use on the hair, there are shampoos with rosemary essences added to help prevent hair loss, which is sometimes common during menopause.

• **Warning.** Shouldn't be used in cases of high blood pressure.

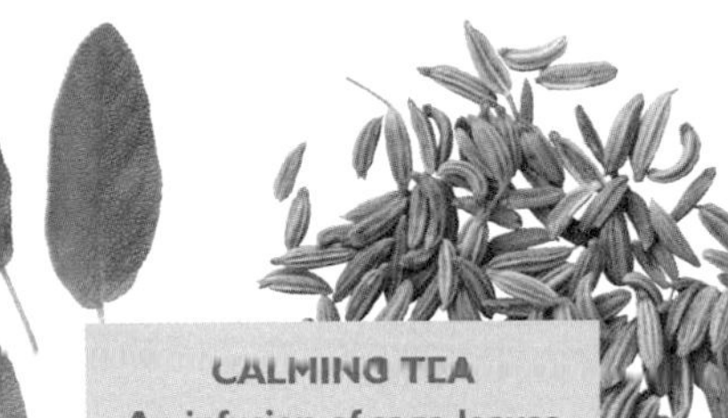

CALMING TEA
An infusion of sage leaves and fennel seeds helps to relieve sore breasts.

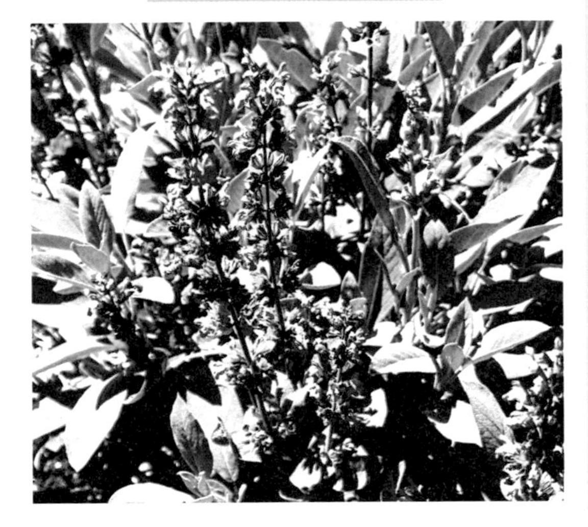

Sage
(Salvia officinalis)

- **Parts used.** The leaves are used to make infusions.
- Although it's native to the Mediterranean it's cultivated in many countries throughout the world.
- It helps blood circulation and stimulates digestion. In the reproductive system it acts as an emmenagogue, provoking menstrual periods; during menopause it can be taken to relieve hot flashes (especially in the hands) and to balance hormonal changes.
- **Warning.** Do not take during pregnancy.

ESSENTIAL OILS FROM A TO Z

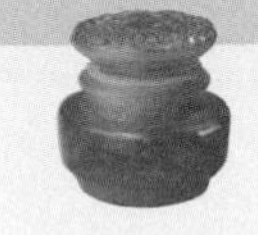

VETIVER
Fights insomnia, depression and anxiety. Strengthens red blood cells, stimulates oxygen flow in the body and tones the reproductive system. Blends well with myrrh, geranium, lavender, rose, sandalwood, ylang ylang. It can be used pure, because it isn't toxic and doesn't irritate the skin.

YLANG YLANG
Reduces blood pressure and relaxes the nervous system.
It also helps to regulate the body's hormonal function and aids in fighting postpartum depression. Blends with lavender, lemon, rose, rosewood and sandalwood.
Safety. Should not be used on inflamed skin or if you suffer from dermatitis. If used excessively, it can cause headaches and nausea.

Feminine caring foods

A balanced diet is the key stone for good health. Increasing consumption of essential fatty acids and the amounts of vitamins and minerals in the daily diet may help to relieve many of the discomforts suffered by women.

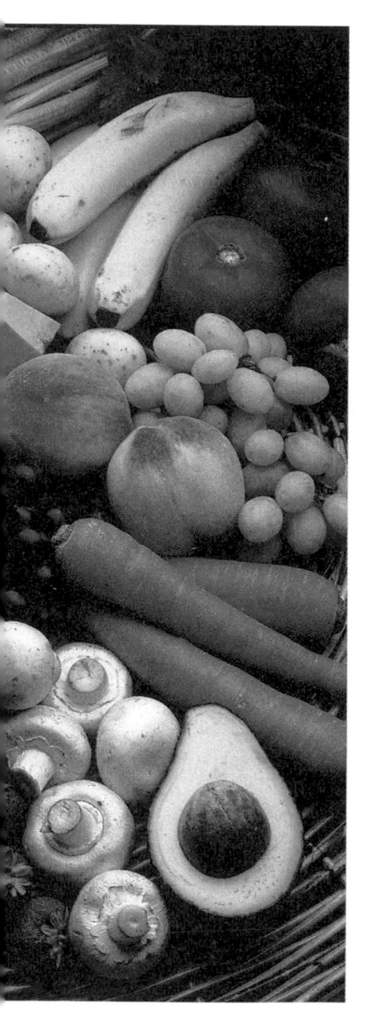

The following foods should be found in a healthy feminine diet.

- **Soy.** And a number of derivatives containing vegetable estrogens that can reduce the risk of heart diseases, osteoporosis and female cancers. Calcium enriched soy products are the best choice.

- **Dairy products.** Low-fat milk, yogurt and reduced fat cheeses are high in calcium and help to reduce the risk of osteoporosis after menopause. Because calcium is found in the liquid part of milk, extracting fat from dairy products doesn't reduce the mineral content.

- **Whole foods.** Rich in insoluble fiber, breads and whole grains are basic low fat sources of energy that reduce the risk of breast and uterine cancer. They also help to prevent colon cancer, flushing the intestines and improving waste flow.

- **Berries.** Rich in fito-nutrients, red, black and blueberries help to strengthen collagen production, the

FIGHTING CANDIDIASIS

Candida albicans is a yeast present in the intestines and in general doesn't have any adverse effects. It only becomes a problem when it grows rapidly and excessively. This can occur in the intestine and in the vagina, but also in the mouth and throat. The most important key in preventing it, is to strengthen the immune system. You may want to try the following foods:

- **Garlic**, which helps to prevent viral, bacterial and yeast infections, increasing the resistance of the immune system.

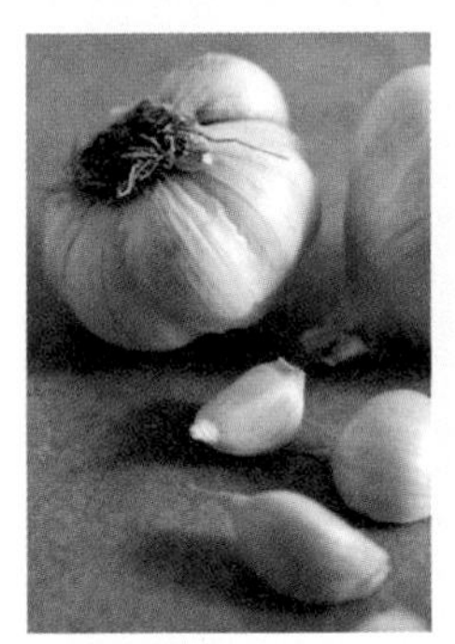

- **Foods rich in zinc** such as red **meat**, **fish**, **dried fruits**, **seeds** and **dairy products**, especially **yogurt**.
- Fruit drinks that contain **"probiotic"** bacteria that help to restore the balance of microorganisms in the intestines that keep candida under control. Yogurt is also good.
- **Iron rich food**s, like **lentils**. An iron deficiency can induce the growth of candida.
- **Grapefruit seed extract**, called "citricidal" is recommended to treat candidiasis for its powerful anti-mycotic effects and its ability to keep intact beneficial bacteria inside the intestines.

It's also advised to avoid excess sugar which can create a stock pool for candida to feed on. Diabetics tend to suffer from this vaginal yeast infection regularly.

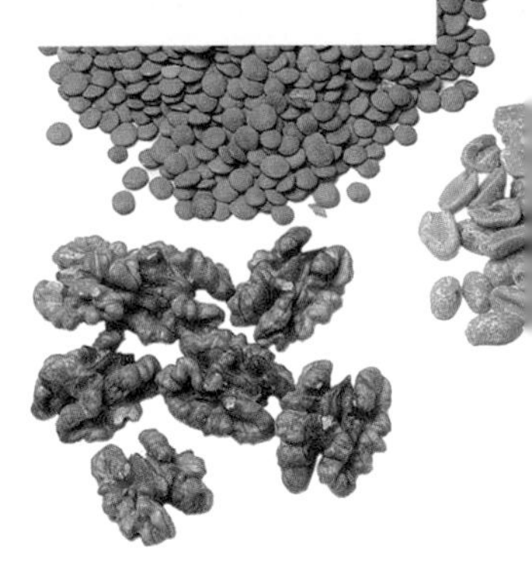

artery walls and the proteins that make up the skin's structure and volume. Help to reverse visible signs of aging.

- **Fish, dried fruits and seeds.** Rich in essential fatty-acids, necessary for keeping the cells hydrated (lack of these essential fatty-acids can cause the skin to dry out). Ocean fish are rich in iron that the body can absorb easily.

- **Lean red meat.** Reduces the risk of anaemia and provides minerals that are necessary for the health of the reproductive system.

NOTE
You should always consult your doctor before changing your diet.

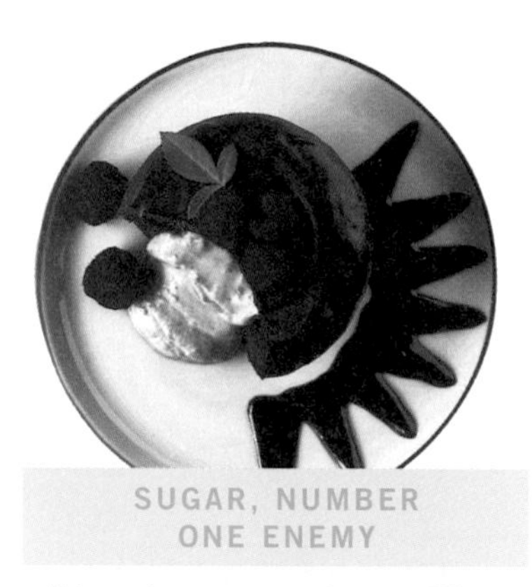

SUGAR, NUMBER ONE ENEMY

Women's great enemy is sugar. Often, in the face of fatigue, tiredness or depression we feel an impulse to eat sweets but the end effect of eating sugars is a drop in blood sugar levels, making us feel more tired or increase depression. This is also generated by the hormonal mechanism: when we eat sweets the pancreas reacts to the increase of sugar in the blood and releases a large amount of insulin. This causes a rapid decline in blood sugar levels and produces hypoglycemia. What is the consequence? Increased fatigue, tiredness and depression. It is important especially during your menstrual periods to keep a balanced level of sugar in the blood.

It is recommended during menstruation, when you feel tired or have an irresistible craving to eat something sweet, eat some honey. At the same time excess refined sugar modifies the pH in the stomach, which is why the body when trying to balance alkaline levels, takes calcium from the bones, decreasing bone's mineral density.

- **Beets.** Rich in foliate (folic acid), reducing the risk of spinal defects in babies and low levels of red blood cells in the blood.
- **Pears.** Help to reduce cholesterol and regulate sugar levels in the blood.
- **Eggplant.** High in antioxidants and helps to reduce high levels of cholesterol, it also helps to protect the brain.
- **Chickpeas.** Rich in isoflavones that help to reduce the risk of cancers related to hormones and relieve menopause symptoms.
- **Flax seeds.** Rich in fatty acids that can help to relieve PMS.
- **Avocado.** Rich in vitamin E, a necessary vitamin for the skin's health.
- **Black currants.** Rich in vitamin C and a rich source of antioxidants. Reduce the risk of certain cancers and strengthen the immune system.
- **Garlic.** High in fito nutrients and anti mycotic activity. Good for preventing and treating candidiasis.

FOR PREVENTING BREAST CANCER

Breast cancer can be caused by a number of factors.
However, eating a healthy diet is one of the key variables in preventing and reducing the risk of breast cancer.
A nutritional guide has been put together to help prevent breast cancer.
It's important to reduce your intake of **animal** fat present in foods such as **butter**, **creams**, **dairy products**, **deli meats**, **sausages**, **fatty meats** and **poultry skin**.
It's important to eat **fresh**, **raw fruits** and **vegetables** that can benefit the intestinal walls, prevent constipation, an important factor in reducing the risk of any health problem.
In the case of cancer, a healthy intestinal wall increases the body's defenses and stops the cells from mutating. Fiber plays a key role in preventing cancer, flushing out free radicals and the detoxification of many xenobiotics that when they come into contact with the intestinal mucous can cause dangerous mutations. This is why whole foods included in the diet can be extremely helpful.

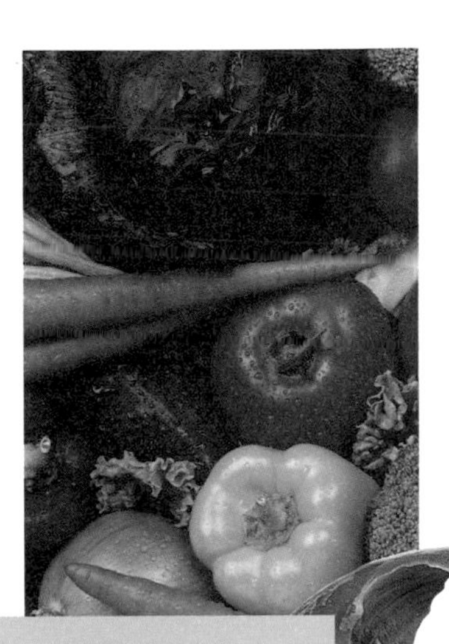

KEY NUTRITION

- **Eat raw fruit and vegetables daily to increase your intake of fibers.**
- **Decrease fatty meats and whole milk dairy products.**
- **Eat soy at least two times per week, to replace meat. You can eat soybeans or derived products (burgers, tofu, soy milk, miso and many other products), preferably organic.**
- **Increase the amount of beans and flaxseed in your diet. They contain phytoestrogens that reduce the risk of many discomforts caused by the hormonal metabolism.**
- **Make sure to eat many antioxidant rich foods and to eat plenty of fresh foods and stay away from processed fast foods.**

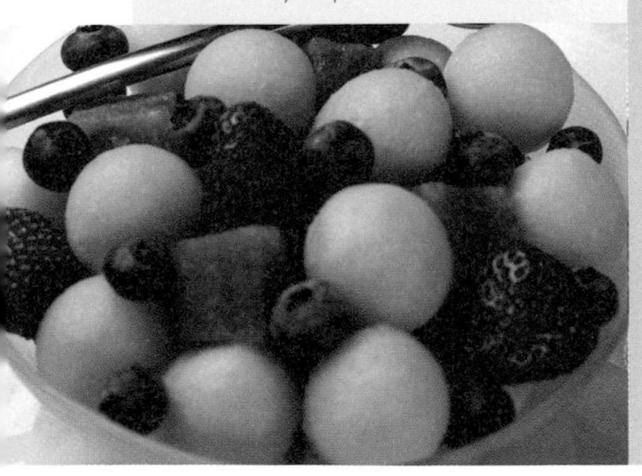

Foods for those "difficult" days

Bothersome PMS symptoms and menstrual pains can be prevented and eliminated with a healthy diet, that includes a balance in essential nutrients and certain foods that fortify the female reproductive system.

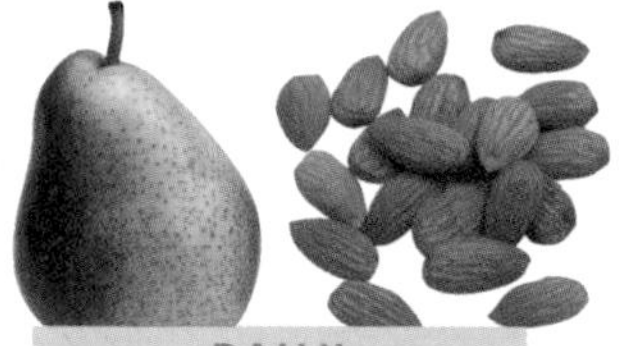

DAILY RECOMMENDATION FOR PMS

Ingredients

1 tablespoon wheat germ,
3 almonds,
1 tablespoon flaxseed.

Preparation

Grind and mix with 1 grated pear or apple or 1 crushed banana.

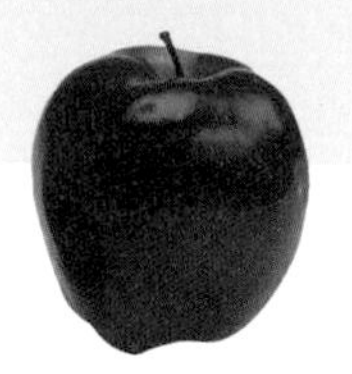

An emotional imbalance brought on by PMS is caused by the alteration in the relative concentrations of estrogens and progesterone. This causes a series of hormonal imbalances, among those a decrease of endorphins in the body. This is why the principle vitamin important for the body is vitamin B_6, especially if you are taking birth control pills, because they increase the need for this vitamin that helps to lower estrogen levels and flush out retained water. Iron, magnesium, zinc and poli-unsaturated fatty acids (those that are found in vegetable oils) are also essential to your diet. It's also recommended to increase the amount of foods high in these nutrients, such as brewer's yeast, and replacing refined flour and grains with whole grains.

- **Vitamin B_6.** Found in **lentils, meats, vegetables** and **dried fruits**.

- **Zinc.** Found in **fresh oysters, sesame seeds, ginger root, wholewheat flour, nuts** and **red meat**.

■ **Magnesium.** Found in **green leafy vegetables, bananas, wheat germ, fish, seaweed** and **dried fruits.**

AGAINST DEPRESSION

Tryptophan is an aminoacid that the body converts into serotonin, a brain chemical that transmits signals. This brain food helps to relieve depression. Turkey and ricotta cheese are rich in the aminoacid tryptophan.

BENEFICIAL FOODS

- **Sunflower seeds**, **pumpkinseeds**, **flaxseed** and **sesame seeds** as well as **hemp oil** are rich in fatty acid Omega-6. Deficiency can aggravate PMS.
- **Rye bread**, **pastas**, **breakfast cereals**, **basmati rice**, **beans** and **fruit** contain sugars that are broken down slowly, and gradually released into the blood stream. This helps to control the anxiety brought on by drops or peaks in blood sugar.
- **Avocado**, **dates**, **bananas**, **plums**, **eggplant**, **pineapple** and **tomatoes** contain serotonin, which is found in some receptor points in the stomach and can cause chain reactions similar to serotonin in the brain, bringing well-being and increased energy.
- **Lentils**, **spinach**, **chickpeas**, **fish**, **lean meats**, **enriched milk**, **amaranth** and **millet** are iron rich foods, a fundamental mineral during menstruation.

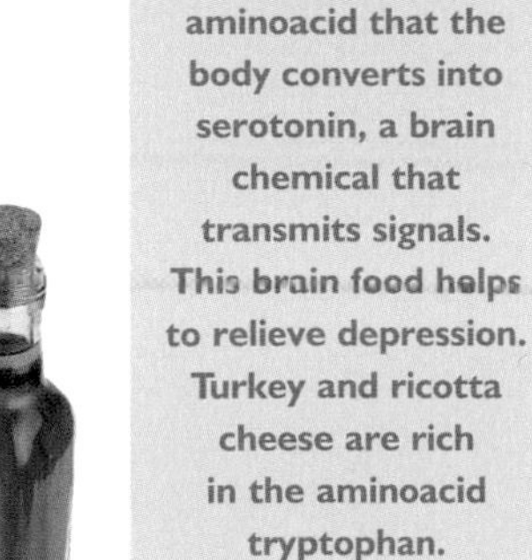

FOODS TO AVOID

- **Meat products**, **cakes** and **cookies**, **whole milk products** and **salty foods cooked in saturated fats** should be avoided, because they can interfere with the metabolism of fatty acids Omega-6 and cause weight gain.
- **Coffee**, **tea**, **cola drinks** and **pain relievers** contain caffeine which stimulates the nervous system and can worsen symptoms like irritability.
- **Prepackages** or **canned foods** are high in sodium, making you retain liquids.

Foods during pregnancy

A balanced diet and keeping the mother healthy during conception and throughout pregnancy are crucial for a baby's growth in the uterus. Here's a recommended diet for future mommy and baby.

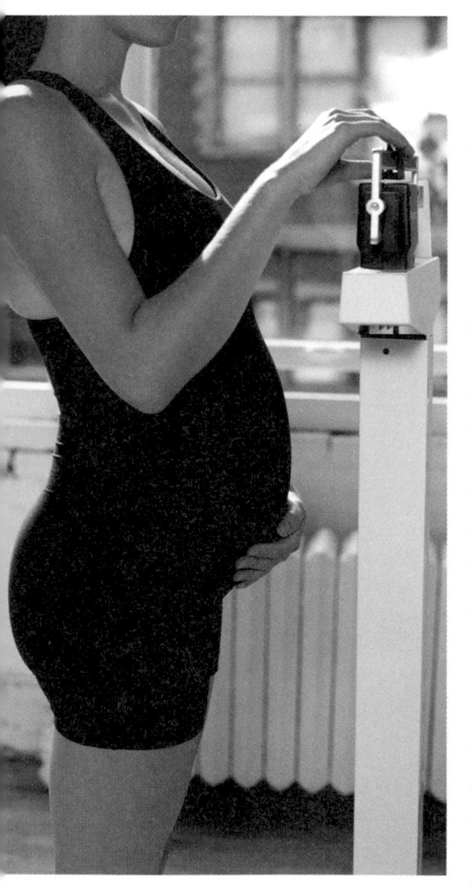

During pregnancy women's bodies use up more energy, increasing the rate of metabolism, which makes a higher calorie intake necessary. A pregnant woman needs around 300 more calories a day than a normal diet. It's advised that you eat smaller meals, several times a day: five or six light meals a day that are rich in nutrients is better than one or two heavy meals a day.

TAKE ADVANTAGE OF FOOD VALUES

To optimize the absorption of nutrients:

- Eat organic foods, avoid preservatives and additives.
- Eat fresh and raw foods whenever possible. Steam foods instead of boiling and avoid fried foods.
- Drink filtered water and wash all fruits and vegetables.
- Avoid excess salt that can cause water retention, especially in the legs. For the same reason don't drink too much mineral water.
- Many nutrients act in synergy with other

nutrients, which is why it's recommended to take a multi-vitamin and mineral supplement rather than taking vitamins and minerals separately. Consult your doctor.

- Eat a wide range of foods that include all essential nutrients.

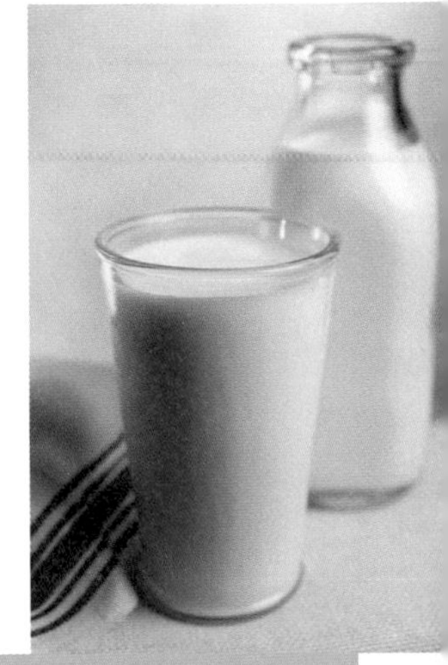

ANTI-NUTRIENTS

These foods inhibit the absorption of nutrients causing a negative balance in the nutritional level. Some foods you should remove from your diet:

- Do not drink alcohol. It can harm the baby and impedes the body from absorbing vitamin B, calcium, iron, zinc and magnesium. It also increases blood pressure.
- Don't smoke. Cigarette smoke (first and second hand) can cause miscarriage, birth defects, premature birth and low birth weight. It also reduces the amount of oxygen and nutrients for the fetus. Nicotine increases the reduction of calcium and destroys vitamin C.
- Avoid tea and coffee that tend to have a diuretic effect that can interfere with the absorption of calcium, magnesium, zinc and iron.
- Don't take strong laxatives because they can weaken the fetus and the uterus.

ESSENTIAL NUTRIENTS AND THEIR SOURCES

- **Calcium.** Low fat milk, cheese, yogurt, beans, eggs, tofu and whole grains.
- **Iron.** Red meat and poultry, dark fish, beans, shellfish, fortified grains, nuts, seeds, dried fruits, dark green leafy vegetables.
- **Zinc.** Red meat and poultry, oysters and other shellfish, beans, kiwi.
- **Vitamin B (includes foliate).** Red meat and poultry, fish, dairy products, fortified cereals, nuts, seeds, dark green leafy vegetables, beans, orange juice, bananas, avocado, whole grains.
- **Vitamin C.** Citrus fruit, tomatoes, red peppers, strawberries, kiwi, parsley.
- **Potassium.** Figs, plumbs, raisins, bananas, broccoli, cauliflower, mushrooms, sweet potatoes, tomatoes.

A DIET FOR EACH TRIMESTER

During each stage of pregnancy women have different nutritional needs. A food guide for each of the three trimesters, and an example of one day healthy diet have been put together for you.

First trimester

During the first trimester it's not necessary to increase the amount of food you eat. A diverse diet rich in lean meats, fruit, vegetables and dairy is enough. The pregnant woman needs proteins to develop and repair cells, muscles, organs, tissue, hair and for the production of enzymes. She also needs foliate (a B vitamin used in cell division, the formation of red blood cells and to build the nervous system of the newborn) and iron (essential mineral to transport oxygen and to produce energy).

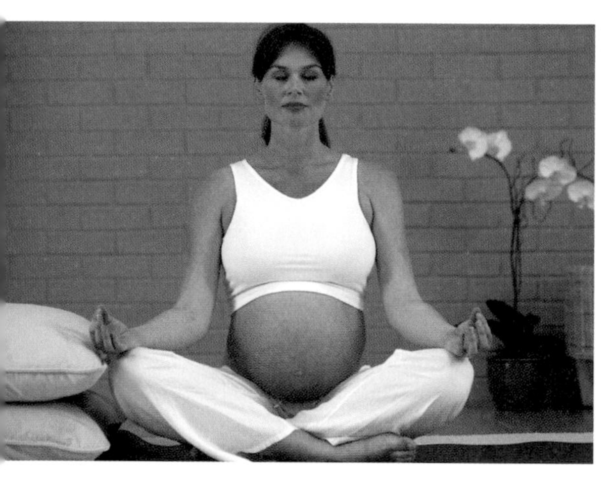

1st TRIMESTER

BREAKFAST *Fortified oatmeal with banana, pear and milk.*	**SNACK** *1 slice of oatmeal cake with almonds and 1 fruit smoothy.*
MID-MORNING SNACK *1 yogurt and 1 apple.*	**DINNER** *Vegetable tart; tomato, mozzarella and basil salad; dried figs.*
LUNCH *Fish with mashed pumpkin or squash and steamed spinach; 1 tomato; 1 slice of wholewheat bread; 1 orange.*	**BED-TIME REFRESHMENT** *1 slice of wholewheat bread with blackberry jam and cream cheese.*

Second trimester

Key nutrients include calcium (for the baby's formation of strong bones, teeth and muscle growth), phosphorus (for the baby's bones and teeth and to provide energy for mommy and baby and for breast milk) and magnesium (for the baby's liver and heart function and for proper metabolism of proteins and carbohydrates).

In the third trimester

The baby's brain grows faster then even. Essential fathy acids, Omega-6 and Omega-3, are fundamentally important for the brain to function well. The best dietary sources of Omega-6 are **seeds** and **their oils**. The best sources of Omega-3 are **flax seeds, pumpkin** or **squash** and **fish**.

2nd TRIMESTER

BREAKFAST
Cereal with sunflower seeds, banana and milk; 1 bread toasted; orange juice.

MID-MORNING SNACK
1 yogurt with hazelnuts and plums.

LUNCH
Avocado and salmon sandwich on wholewheat bread; 1 kiwi and 1 slice of melon.

SNACK
1 piece of apple pie or cheese cake.

DINNER
Roasted lamb with peas, potatoes, carrots and broccoli. 1 fruit.

BED-TIME REFRESHMENT
Popcorn; 1 glass of warm milk.

3rd TRIMESTER

BREAKFAST
Wheat bran with raisins and milk; grapefruit juice; sardines or fresh grilled tuna and tomatoes on a piece of toast.

MID-MORNING SNACK
Fruit and milk smoothy

LUNCH
Broccoli soup with sunflower seeds; Turkey, spinach and barley sandwich on wholewheat bread; 1 kiwi and 1 slice of melon.

SNACK
Peach and orange smoothy with yogurt. 10 Brazil nuts; 1 slice of watermelon.

DINNER
Chicken and vegetable stir-fry with broccoli, soy sprouts, ginger, whole grain corn, lentil, and potatoes.

BED-TIME SNACK
Tomato soup, 1 slice of wholewheat bread with cream cheese and 2 slices of avocado.

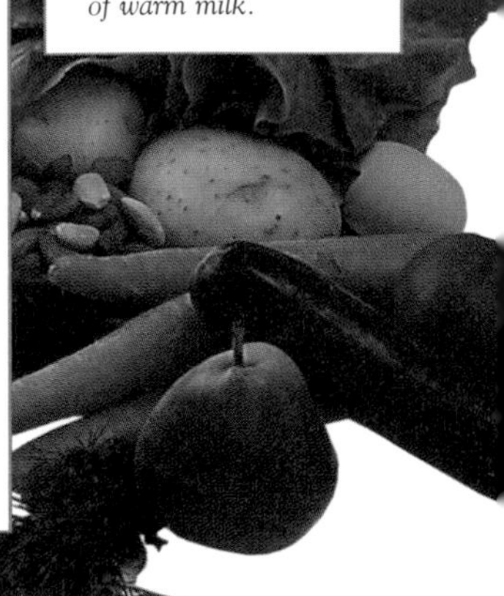

Foods for menopause

When we reach 50 our production of estrogen and progesterone lowers and most women have their last menstrual cycle. These changes can present a number of effects; changes in mood, hot flashes, anxiety and other symptoms. A few keys in getting over symptoms can be in a healthy and nutritionally balanced diet.

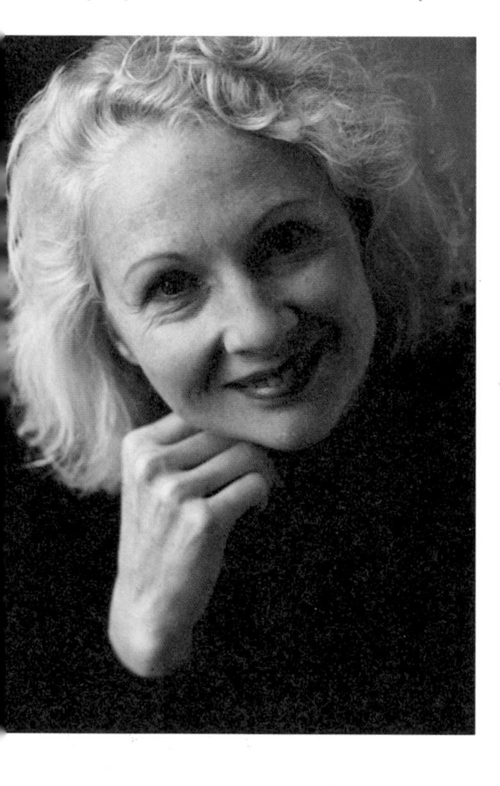

FOLIC ACID
Enriched bread, breakfast cereals and brewer's yeast are excellent sources of folic acid, a B vitamin, that studies have shown reduces the risk of heart diseases.

✚ A healthy and balanced diet can be useful in relieving a number of discomforts brought on by menopause.

- **Soy products** and **soy** are rich in vegetable estrogen. Studies have shown that a diet with ample amounts of soy can reduce hot flashes, vaginal drying and loss in bone density, as well as reducing cholesterol in the blood.
- **Seeds** and **alfalfa sprouts, flaxseeds** and **red clover** also are rich in vegetable estrogen, helping to reduce the thinning of vaginal tissue.
- **Broccoli, barley, cauliflower** and **cabbage** contain phytonutrients that increase the activity of estrogen. It also helps to maintain the flexibility in the skin, artery walls, capillaries and protects

SARDINES
Sardines in brine and eaten whole are a great source of calcium. In addition they are rich in vitamin D and fatty acids Omega-3, that improve the absorption of calcium and reduce the flushing out of nutrients in urine and fecal matter.

the blood vessels that provide oxygen, preventing the risk of heart diseases.

- **Oranges**, grapefruits, **berries, papayas, salad greens, peppers**, sweet **potatoes** and **potatoes** are rich in vitamin C. **Avocados, whole grains, dried fruits** and **seeds** are rich in vitamin E. These two vitamins are antioxidants that can help to protect the skin and keep it firm, at the same time protecting the organs against degenerative diseases.

- **Beets, chickpeas, brussels sprouts, asparagus, peas, green beans** and **sprouts** are rich sources of foliate, the way to incorporate folic acid into your diet.

- **Garlic** is a sulfur rich food that helps to reduce cholesterol and reduce the risk of heart diseases.

- **Ocean fish**, such as **cod, salmon, sardines** and **herring** protect the body against heart disease and are calcium rich foods that should be included in the diet.

- **Red wine** is a source of phytoestrogens. Obviously, drink wine in moderation; no more than a glass (50-80 ml) per meal. It also acts as an antioxidant.

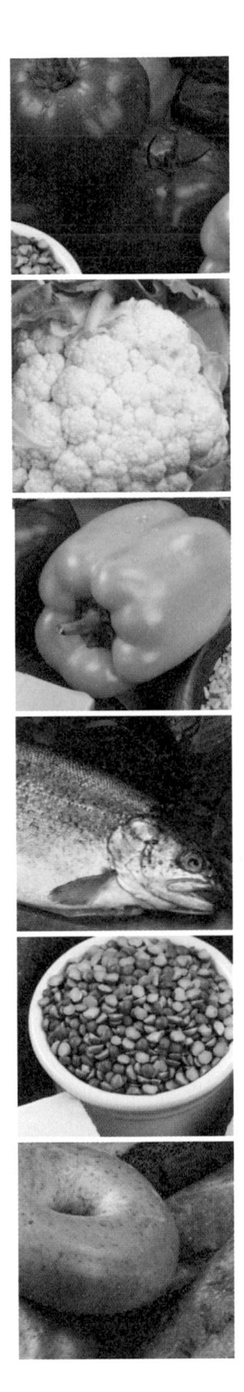

index

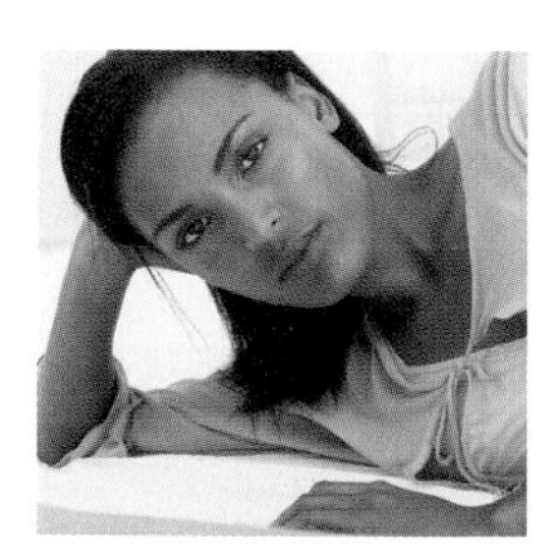